EXTENSION
of
LIFE

Self - Healing

Don't let your time run out.

Michael Sienkiewicz

Reverse your aging process now !

ISBN: 1-4392-4114-7
ISBN-13: 9781439241141

Visit www.booksurge.com to order additional copies.

Acknowledgment

I would like to thank the following people for helping me edit my book Joe Cail, Bill Bambrick, my lovely wife Wendy, Jeff Barnett, and my daughter Brenda lee Sienkiewicz for the pictures throughout the book.

EXTENSION *of* LIFE: *Self Healing*

Includes Reversing Arterial and Cardiovascular Aging, Blood Testing Results, Diet, Supplement, Immune System, Cure Prostate Cancer, Prevent Erectile Dysfunction, Prevent Multiple Sclerosis, Prevent Alzheimer's, Glycosylation, Bone Density, Sports Physiology, Stem Cell Regeneration, and Restless Leg Syndrome.

— *Michael Sienkiewicz*

Disclaimer

There is one very important caution I must stress at the outset of this book. Before beginning any regimen of physical therapy, you must absolutely and positively consult your physician. There may be something else, besides normal aging, that is causing your pain or other symptoms, and only your doctor can tell whether you should be engaging in any of my procedures mentioned in this book. A doctor could also explain what I am recommending or ask for a clarification. If you are otherwise healthy, I'm sure your doctor will agree that it is good, sound therapy. But you may need other treatments as well, and only a licensed physician can provide that. You must know that everything I say in this book is simply my opinion. If you do anything I recommend without the supervision of a licensed medical doctor, you do so at your own risk. I am not making an attempt to prescribe any medical treatment, since under the laws of the United States, only a licensed medical doctor can do so. This book is only my opinions, my thoughts, and my conclusions.

Part 1

Deep Massage and Flexing
Regeneration of Muscle Mass

Part 2

Aging And Health Are Reversible Through Your Diet

Introduction

Who wouldn't give practically anything to be able to rejuvenate his or her body in the golden years of life: To literally reverse the inevitable aging process we all have to endure? I know the answer: Who wouldn't! That, in a nutshell, is what this book is about. Now, don't get me wrong, there is nothing on God's green earth that is going to give you immortality. But, I am going to show you ways that will enable you to live much longer than you ever thought possible, and to live without the pain and discomfort you thought were inevitable.

It wouldn't be unusual for anyone reading this claim to be a little skeptical. So rest assured that what you will read here is based on my own personal experience and a lot of knowledge accumulated over many years. I have put the techniques I am going to share with you into practice, and I am here to tell you that they work. At the age of sixty-six I feel and perform like a 40-year-old.

What you will learn in this book is how to control your systems so that they work in your favor, to create a better life. The great thing is that it's never too early or too late to start making these changes. You don't need a complete overhaul, because, frankly, your body is a pretty fine piece of machinery. What you'll ultimately do is find and fix your own personal weak links. The things that make you most vulnerable to the effects of aging. By restricting calories, increasing your strength, and getting quality sleep are three of nature's best anti-aging medicines. Wouldn't you want to hold the power of your future in your hands, rather than put it in someone else's? Just because you've made mistakes in the past doesn't mean you can't reverse them. No matter what kind of life you've already led, aging is reversible. You can have a do-over if you want it. If you perform a good habit for three years, the effect on your body is as if you've done it your entire life. Even better, within three months of changing a behavior, you can start to measure a difference in your life expectancy. As I said, aging is inevitable, but the rate of aging is not. After all, living longer shouldn't be about taking longer to die. It should be about enjoying every moment of a longer life. You don't want to grow old. You want to stay young.

The other day I was talking to my wife about the idea of writing this book. She asked me: "What makes you think you have the special training necessary to write this book?" I reminded her that I have made a discovery that is unique among mankind: I am the only person I know of who can claim to have found the way to reverse the aging process. Just six years ago, at the age of sixty, I found myself feeling truly old, with all the usual problems of the aged. I could no longer run like I used to. Even walking was painful due to my sore feet. I didn't feel healthy at all: My muscle tone was shot, I felt weak and run-down, my body looked old, I had a prostate problem, high cholesterol, high blood pressure, and serious problems with my internal plumbing. However in just six short years all these symptoms had changed for the better. Today I feel like I am forty years old, enjoying the best of health. All these results were obtained with a healthy diet and using flexing and massaging.

Every day I am bombarded with radio and commercials ads from practitioners claiming they have found the secret of youth: That they have discovered how to reverse the aging process and restore you to youthful vigor. When I examined their methods I found that they were using steroids and growth hormones in small quantities, and their patients were willing to part with thousands of dollars a year. All this without knowing about the potential side effect of these drugs.

Your own body produces its own steroids and growth hormones. But your body needs to be stimulated in the correct way to have it produce these chemicals. I have discovered a way to coax your body into producing them. I have found a way to stimulate and tax the muscle which will increase the rate of growth hormone secretion. Growth hormone in turn, promotes synthesis of new protein while at the same time conserving the proteins already present in the cell causing the muscle to grow. The precise mechanisms that control secretion of growth hormone are not fully understood but stimulation (stress) is known to stimulate secretion.

Synthesis of almost any chemical compound, in this case new muscle mass, requires energy. For instance, a single protein molecule (muscle) might be composed of as many as several thousand amino acids attached to one another by peptide linkages; the formation of each of this linkages requires energy derived from the breakdown of four high-energy bonds; these, many thousand ATP molecules must release their energy as each protein molecule is formed. Indeed, some cells use as much as 75 percent of all the ATP formed in the cell. Simply to synthesize new chemical compounds, especially protein molecules. More than 95 percent of this

ATP is formed in the mitochondria, which accounts for the mitochondria being called the "power houses" of the cell.

The synthesis of proteins is one of the most energy-consuming processes of the cell. When actively flexing and massaging procedures your body will be producing new protein (muscle) at a very rapid rate. During protein production you will feel tired. While doing flexing and massaging for up to two hours in the evening: I would go to bed at night and wake-up in the morning very tired. My body would be drained of energy from producing new protein. There was an instance when I was tired for two days. I didn't have any energy. I didn't know why until I found an article about protein synthesis. I resolved the problems of being tired by consuming simple carbohydrates. Complex carbohydrates didn't work. During protein synthesis our bodies require extra simple carbohydrates. Simple carbohydrates should not be part of your daily diet unless your goal is to recover energy from protein synthesis.

As you read this book, I will share with you how to make all the following things happen. Some benefits include improved muscle tone, increased muscle mass, decreased body fat, increased sex drive, increased bone density and an improved outlook on life. This therapy could change the quality of life for millions of people and change the very nature of our final years.

I am a retired school teacher, with a degree in biology and 33 years of experience teaching science. By the time I reached the age of 60, I was beginning to feel very old. My feet were very painful, causing severe discomfort when I walked. My body's overall muscle tone was to put it mildly, flabby.

I had been unable to run for the previous six years. I would lie in bed at night and think to myself, "This is it, Mike. You're on the downward plunge into that great abyss". I realized I could die at any time and the thought was frightening. I was much too young to let go. So I started to search for ways to prevent that plunge.

My first step was to splurge on a copy of the best book available on human physiology; a 1400-page textbook entitled *Medical Physiology*. This textbook taught me everything I needed to know about how the body works. It is the same book used nationwide in medical schools today. I discovered a wealth of knowledge about my body and how it works. The human body is a magnificent machine, able to do amazing things. But it has to be given a chance, just like any complex machine.

Medical Physiology explained that the human body ought to be able to live up to 150 years. So I have 86 more years to live! And if I feel and stay healthy, I can enjoy those 86 years to the fullest. The father of gerontology (aging research) believes humans could live to 1,000-forever youthful and disease free. The National Institute of Health is funding aging related medicine with an annual budget to around $3 billion. This proves what I'm doing is not make believe.

Aubrey de Grey (father of gerontology) is on a crusade. The British biologist, whose life-extension theories are turning the sluggish field of gerontology on its balding head. He is determined to reinvent human aging by doing away with it altogether. Grey said "aging kills 100,000 people a day. There is a moral obligation to combat this disease. Aging is just the same." I believe I have solved this problem. I feel and perform like a forty year old. My body looks very young and is very muscular and only time will tell. I can improve your quality of life and do away with the ache and pain that goes along with it. I have read many articles on gerontology. It is interesting that their research is with lab mice. My results are conducted with a human body (mine).

I thought it might help you understand what is to come if I shared some history with you, and while doing so, I wanted to make a point. I started working out and lifting weights while I was in the 9th grade. I continued my weight-lifting regimen all through my early life, right up until I was 55 years old. It was not an idle pursuit and I went at it quite seriously.

Here comes point one: Even though I was continuing to work out regularly, between the ages of 45 and 55 years, I was aware that my body was gradually aging. I could feel the aging process at work, gradually shutting down my systems. I had thought that with this continuous exercise program, my body would stay healthy and vigorous. But at last, this was not the case. The workouts helped, of course, but my body kept aging.

I happened upon a fascinating medical article in which the writer stated that the human body reaches its peak in physical condition at about 30 years of age. There is a slight difference between the sexes: Males reach their peak at about 28 years of age, whereas females peak a little later, at about 33. Every ten years the body's muscle mass declines by about 3 to 6 percent. This is what is known as the "normal aging process". Suddenly I knew why my body was declining.

I learned that fifty percent of the body is muscle mass. As it ages, some of the muscle tissue shrinks and is replaced by fat tissue and fiber. The rate of muscle tissue loss is from three to six percent every ten years and the percentage can be greater if you don't maintain some kind of health care. This is part of the normal aging process the article talked about. It occurred to me that there ought to be a way to reverse that process, to actually stop the shrinkage of muscle tissue. Then, I might be able to stop the aging process in its tracks. Now, that is an idea worth pursuing!

That is exactly what happened to me. I discovered a way to halt this unwelcome aging process, and to actually reverse it. I discovered a way to begin shedding years of declining performance. Impossible though it seems, I found a way to return to the vigor of my forties, by regaining my muscle mass. And, with that came the mental attitude that goes with being younger.

Today, at 66 years of age, I feel like I have shed twenty-five years. I am able to do things I haven't been able to do since I was in my forties. My feet no longer ache, my muscle tone is back to normal - normal for a man in his forties - and, wonder of wonders, I have started to run again. And more to the point, I no longer have those feelings of impending death.

I thought it might be worthwhile to share this with you, in the hope that it would enable you to achieve the same benefits.

As you read this book, I will explain how you, too, can stop your body from aging, and to actually reverse the aging process. As you might expect, once you have achieved that miracle, you will experience a vastly improved quality of life. Gone will be all the aches and pains that you thought were the unavoidable consequences of growing older.

In the rest of the book I will take you on a tour of your body, and explain the concepts for relieving pain and tension that I have learned from personal experimentation. Using these techniques I have been able to transform my body from its former weak condition to the vibrant health I enjoy today in just six years. If things keep going the way they are, I fully expect to live way past the age of one hundred.

The first chapter begins with the feet. Methods for flexing and massaging the various parts of the feet to relieve pain and tension are explained, and the concept known as reflexology is introduced. Subsequent chapters look at the calves, upper legs, the hands, forearms, upper arms, neck, shoulders, back, abdomen, and chest. Special attention is given to massaging the facial muscles, which may be of special interest to women in preventing the sagging that often accompanies aging. Closing chapters will deal with reverse arterial and cardiovascular aging, nutritious diet, including foods which protect your body and food supplements your body needs. I will discuss immune system, prostate cancer, erectile dysfunction, Alzheimer's, glycosylation, multiple sclerosis, restless leg syndrome and sport physiology. Finally, I will discuss how different drugs affect your body.

On Sept 24 2008, I had body composition analysis and bone density test done on my own body and the results were amazing. I have the lean body mass of a 40 year old and the bone density of a 30 year old. All this was made possible through flexing and massaging, by having a good diet and taking the right supplements. All these results can be achieved by reading "EXTENSION OF LIFE":Self Healing.

I spend hundreds of hours doing research and everything in this book is sound medical advice. The materials used are articles that I read and obtained from medical sources. This might not be stated in certain articles that you read. But all information came from sound medical sources. This is the information I used to make myself a youthful healthy adult; with a lean body mass of a 40 year old and bone density of a 30 year old. The material on flexing and massaging are from actual experiments that I performed on my own body. Some of these results were explained with medical information.

THIS IS THE ONLY PROCEDURE THAT CAN REGENER-ATE NEW MUSCLE MASS AND REVERSE THE AGING PROCESS. Enjoy the reading "EXTENSION OF LIFE": Self Healing.

You might think that flexing and massaging will only work for me. How do I know it will work for someone else?

Example one: I spoke to an associate; I'll call him Greg, about my process of creating more muscle mass by flexing and massaging. He asked "How do you know this will work for someone else? Maybe it just works for you." Time went by and I didn't see Greg for a month. When I did see him, he said "flexing and massaging really works. It's like lifting weights." In the month when we didn't see each other, he massaged one pectorals muscle (chest muscle). The muscle became more muscular and increased in size. The other side remained the same as it had been.

Example two: My 42 year old son decided to try flexing and massaging on his biceps. His biceps muscles increased in mass. These are two examples on how flexing and massaging can work for you.

As you read this book, you must expect that it takes a good deal of time to reverse the aging process. Remember that your body has been aging at a rate of three to six percent each decade, so it's going to take a while to reverse this process. But you can do these procedures I will describe while you're standing, sitting, driving, watching TV, playing cards, or at most any convenient time. Remember to start out slowly (once a day or more): The muscle will become sore. This is a good thing. This means the muscle has been stimulated to grow into more muscle mass.

CHAPTER 1:

Foot Flexing and Massaging

I will begin by talking about the feet. The pain I was experiencing in my feet seemed to be the very foundation of all my other problems. We really don't know how important our feet are until we begin to experience problems walking. By the age of 55, my feet were so painful I had to give up running. It seemed to be a downward spiral. As I continued to age, my feet became worse. I found that when I got up to fetch something after sitting for a period of time, my feet would immediately let me know they were sore. It felt like I was walking on pins and needles. I tried many different things to relieve my foot pain. I spent thousands of dollars to solve this problem. I had a foot operation, bought expensive shoes, orthotic made, and nothing worked. If you read this article and your feet become pain free that in itself is a great benefit.

One day I tried a little experiment. I tried flexing my feet for a few minutes, to see what effect it might have. It seemed to work. I noticed that after the flexing I could walk without pain for a short period of time. So I thought, "What if I was to flex my feet on a regular basis? Perhaps this might make the pain disappear permanently". It was worth a try. So I started flexing my feet throughout the day. (I'll tell you how I did it later.) It worked. After doing this for two and a half years, I had said goodbye to foot pain.

Foot flexing is easy and convenient to do. By flexing the toes up or down and pushing down on the foot with pressure from the leg this will cause muscles in the foot to tighten up which will stimulate the muscles to grow. This will also put pressure on the bones in the foot which will increase the bone density making the foot stronger. Bones can be stimulated to grow with pressure throughout life. These pressures will also strength the ligaments in the foot. You can flex them while you are sitting or standing. I found that it was really easy to do this throughout the day. One caution, however: Foot flexing is not a magical cure for foot pains. It takes time. In my case, it took two and a half years to completely lose my pains. But the good news is that it is not at all difficult. It doesn't interfere with anything you may happen to be doing. Within a few months you will definitely begin to feel better, and after a few years, your feet won't hurt any more. We need to remember, Rome wasn't built in a day. It took 30 to 40 years for your feet to become sore, so it will take a while to get them back to normal. Any time you sit down, just flex your feet. It's really easy.

Muscle flexing just becomes a habit, and it's really easy to do. When you flex your feet, you must begin by determining how often and how long to do this. You have to figure this out on your own. I did this throughout the day and my feet felt better. I flexed my feet three or four hours a day. When the feet become pain free, you can reduce this amount of time. Another way of flexing, when sitting in a chair, place pressure on the toes of each foot and raise the heels of each foot off the floor two or more inches. Keeping the heels off the floor, push down with the legs, adding pressure to each foot. This will also strengthen each foot. By flexing the feet, we are building up the muscle mass which was replaced by the fat and fiber tissues and strengthen the bones and ligament in the foot.

There is another method for stimulating the muscles. That is by massaging them. I would suggest a method which I call deep massage. This stimulates muscle growth and increases bone density. Massaging the feet with pressure will break down the muscle and stimulate it to grow. This will also stimulate the bones and ligaments which will strengthen the foot.

I will begin with the various parts of the feet, beginning with the toes. You will need to spend 30 seconds or more on each toe. Rub and massage your toe all the way from the base to the tip. Use small, circular motions as you work your way up the toe, and then employ long strokes from the base to the tip. Repeat these techniques on each toe remember to apply some pressure when doing this. Also, if your toes curl downward, which is not uncommon; simply push down on each joint. This will straighten out the toes which will stretch the ligaments. Then cup your left hand and form a cup around the toes of the right foot, pull back on the toes to stretch the muscles and ligaments in the foot and calf. Hold the pull for several seconds and repeat the pull four or five times. Then repeat this procedure on the left foot. This will help straighten out your toes. The curling of the toes is called crow's feet. The ligaments in the calf and bottom of the foot tighten up causing the toes to curl down. Pulling back on the toes you can feel the ligaments stretching in the bottom of the foot and calf. My toes still curl down but my feet feel better when I do this. If I knew this at an earlier age I could have prevented this from happening.

Next we move to the top and bottom of each foot. Planting your foot on the floor, place your fingers on top of the foot, massaging the top and sides of the foot with your fingers. Place the right ankle on the left knee, cup the finger of the left hand applying pressure with the figure and massage the sole of the right foot from the toes up to the ankle. Use your knuckles to ripple all around the sole. Then, using your thumbs, apply deep pressure to the sole of your foot. Using your finger and thumb, squeeze around your ankle, the Achilles tendon, and the heel. Repeat this procedure to the left foot.

Alternatively, you can use the heel and other foot, as shown in Figure 1, to massage the top, side, and bottom of the other foot. Each morning before I get out of bed I will massage my feet with this method. I will massage one foot against the other and include all the major parts of the foot. Experiment and you will figure out many different ways to massage the foot with this method. This is what I did.

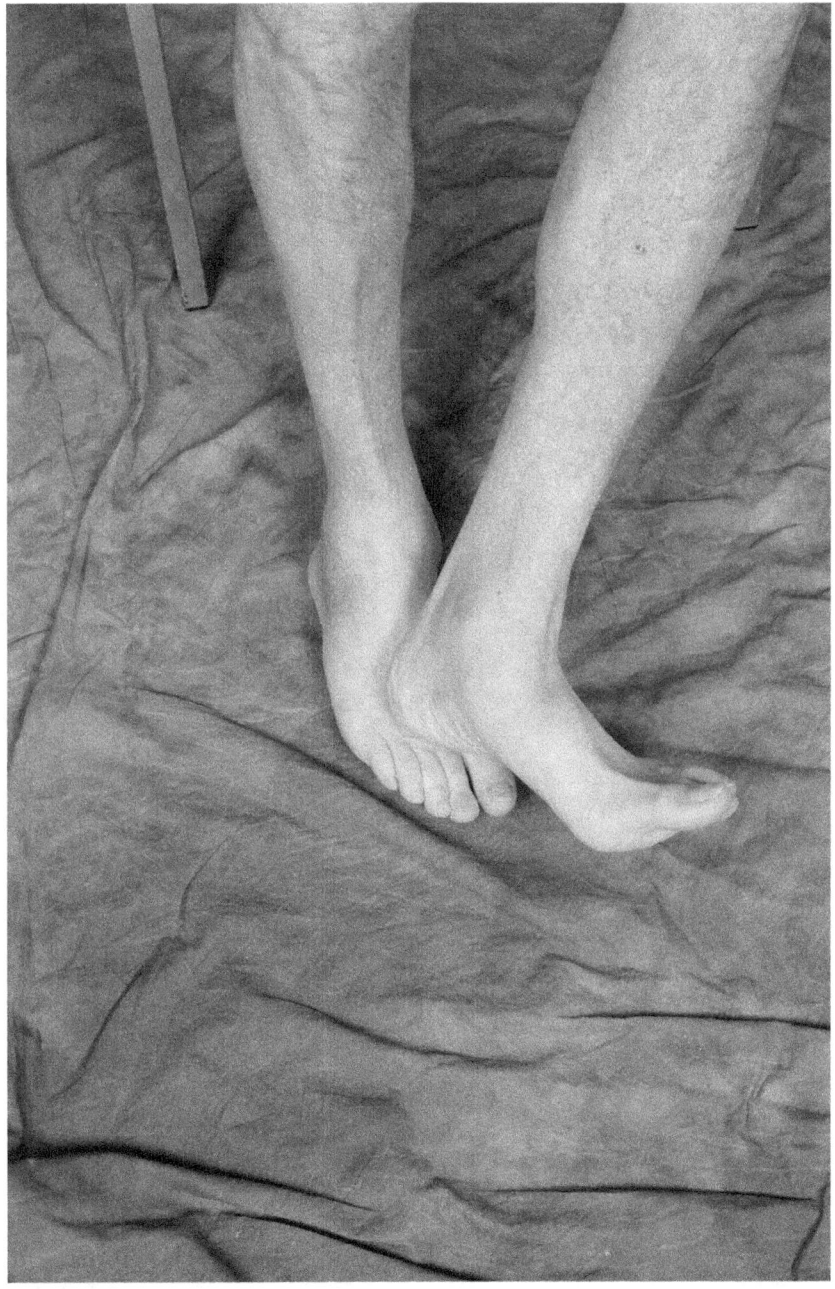

Figure 1: This picture shows the heel foot massage technique.

One convenient way of massaging the sole of the foot is to rub the bottom of one foot against the heel or ankle of the other. Or, you can rub the bottom of the foot against a thick rug or the rung of a coffee table.

Now, take the foot in your hands and gently rotate it laterally at the ankle, first to the right and then the left. Then twist the foot gently from side to side in a rocking motion to loosen up the ankle even more.

Some people find that massaging the foot with a massage stick (Figure 2) is beneficial. This works really well on the arch, sole, and heel of the foot. I message my feet twice a day in the morning and evening.

Figure 2 note the massage sticks are on the top right of photograph, two other types of massage tools and shoes with knobby soles to stimulate the feet.

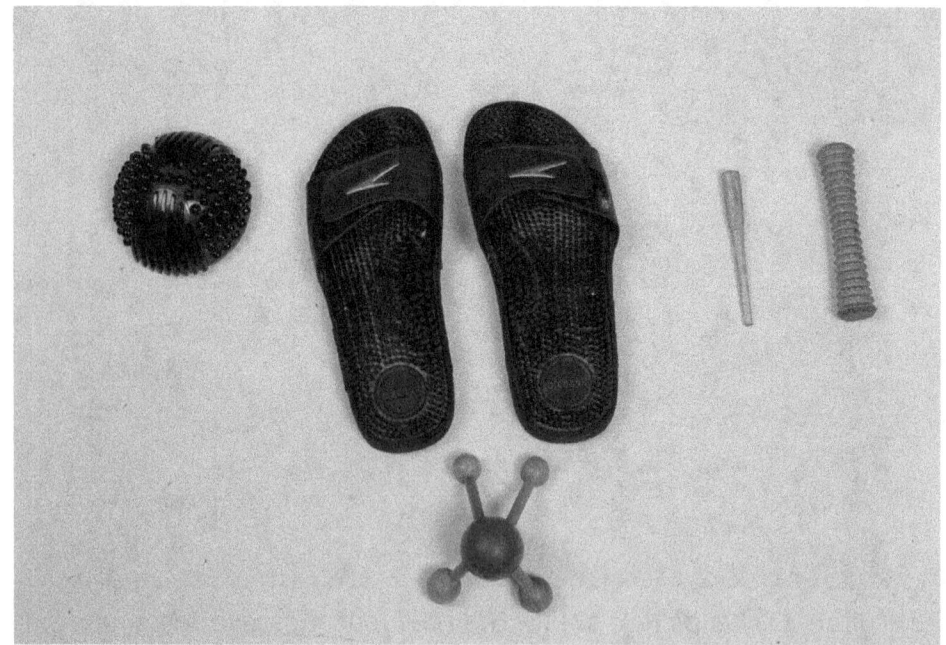

Figure 2

I came across an interesting fact from history. Back in the late forties, Mahatma Gandhi, the Indian leader who espoused passive resistance in his struggle against British rule, used to walk barefoot wherever he journeyed. This was hardly an easy task over the mountainous sections of northern India. At the end of the day, he would have one of his female disciples wash his aching feet, and then she would massage them using a smooth stone. This suggests another very effective way of massaging not only the feet, but all of your muscles. Perhaps you have your own "rock buddy" that could be recruited for the task.

No matter how you do it, flexation and massage will strengthen your feet. Eventually your feet will feel normal again. Remember, it takes time lots of time. It took me two years to rid of my foot pains. The benefits far outweigh the time taken to achieve them.

CHAPTER II:

The Calf

Early in yourself examination, you may discover, as I did, that there are parts of your body that have been causing you pain and discomfort. Perhaps this is even without your knowledge. Some of these problems only show up when you begin to focus on them. I went through this process and concluded that I would have to pay close attention to each major muscle group, working upward from my feet to my head. I couldn't afford to ignore any part of my body - not even the muscles in my face.

Muscles are not a single mass of tissue. They are built up in layers, and each of these layers requires stimulation. Nowhere is this more evident than in the great bunch of muscles in the calf.

Treating the calf muscles demands that you begin massaging the deep layers, proceeding from the top to the bottom. The technique I developed consists of applying pressure with both of the thumbs, as shown in Figure 3. Using a kneading action, work your way all the way down the calf, from top to bottom. Another useful technique is to use your knuckles to do the massaging, as shown in Figure 4. Massage the entire calf in this way, using your knuckles to massage the outer edges and inward to the middle of the calf, over its full length.

After just four months of this massaging, I noticed that my calf muscles were beginning to increase in mass, which was a welcome result, but very surprising to me. I found that deep massage stimulates the muscle, just like lifting weights, causing the calf muscles to increase in size and strength. At the age of 66, my calves are bigger than when I was lifting weights at a much younger age.

It is well known that growth hormones stimulate muscles to grow larger. Since my calves were growing larger in size, this made me wonder if the human body might be capable of producing its own growth hormones. I learned that this is, indeed, the case. The mechanism seems to be the flexing and massaging of the muscle fibers. Apparently this is what we do when we lift weights. I was achieving the same result without the weights. At any rate, the end result, and a most satisfying one, was that I was producing larger, more powerful and more elastic muscles.

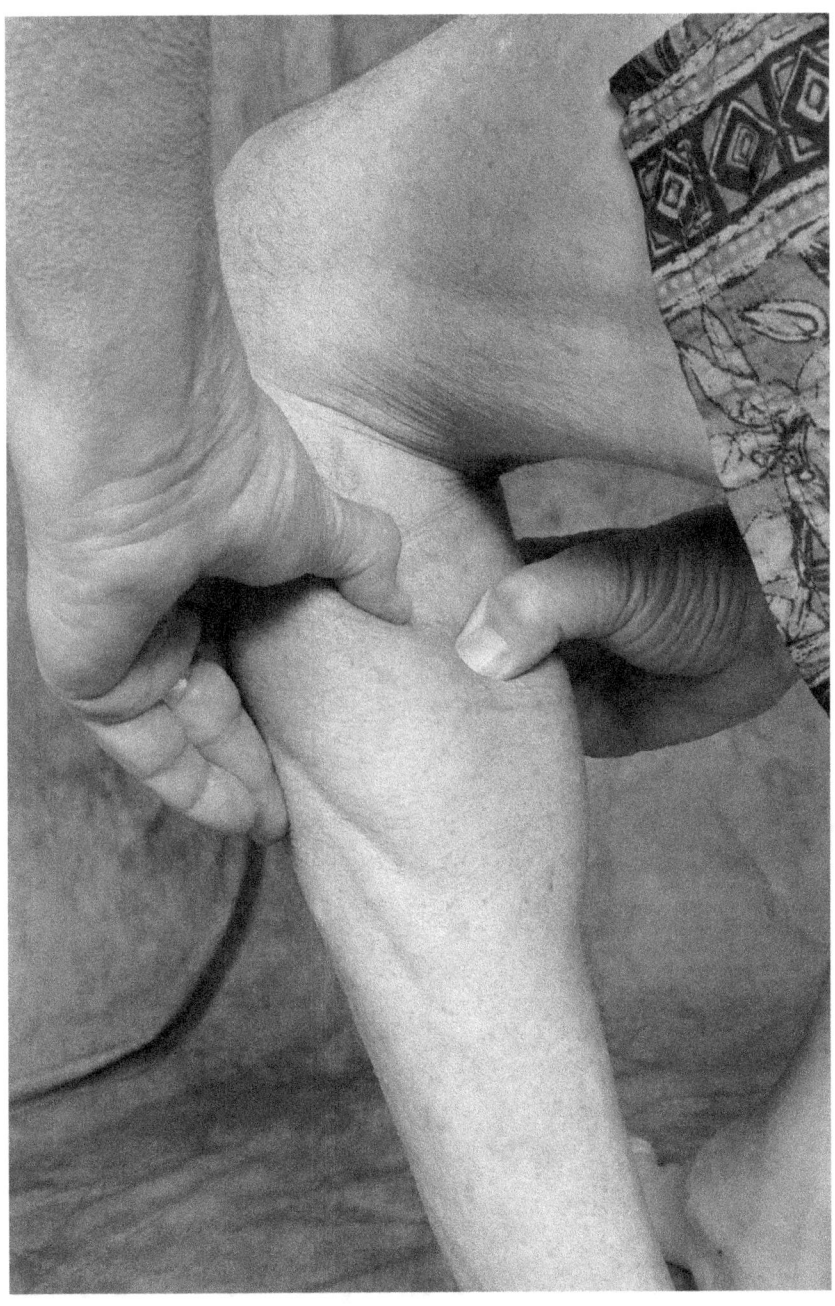

Figure 3: Kneading technique.

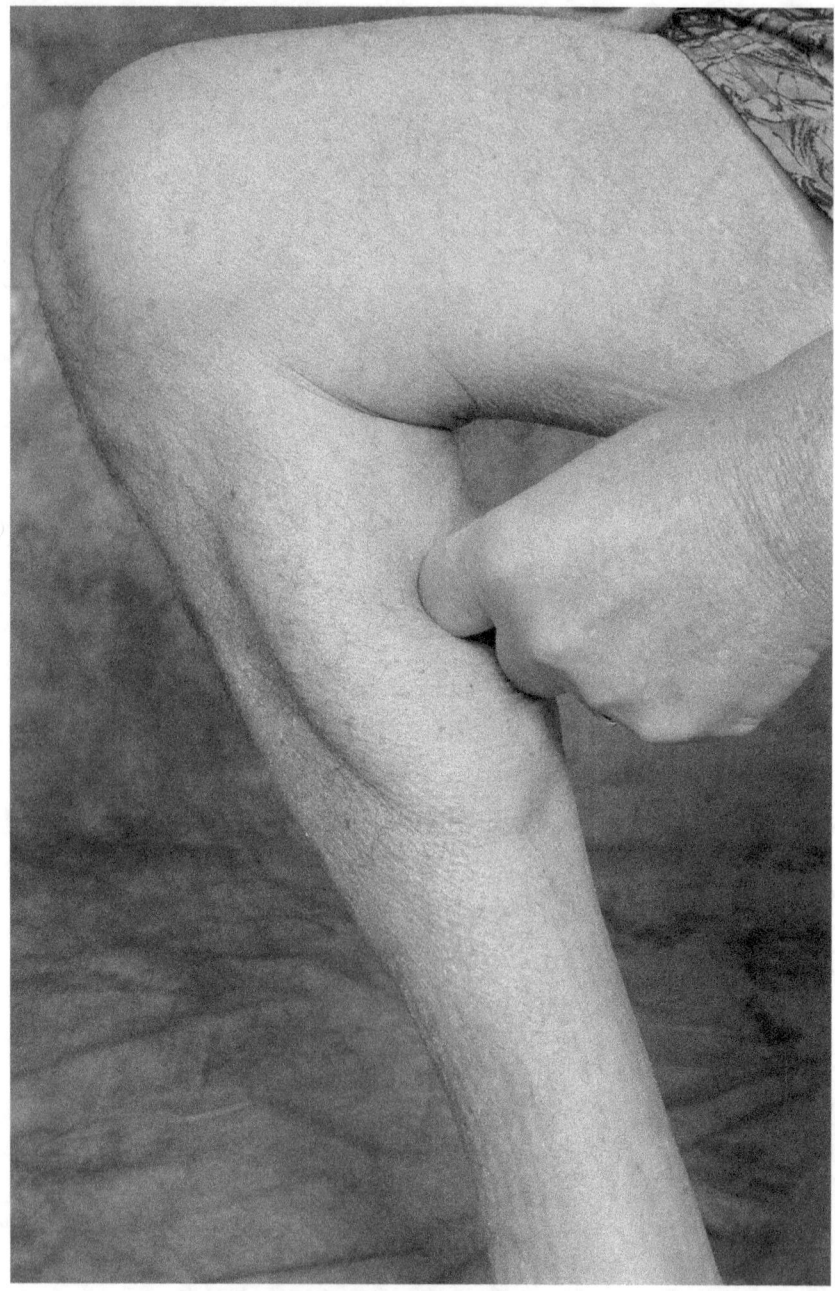

Figure 4: Knuckle massage.

Do not feel limited to the simple methods I have mentioned for stimulating the calf muscles. You can also massage them by placing the calf of one leg atop the knee of the opposite leg, as illustrated in Figure 5. The technique is to slide the calf up and down the knee. You can go all the way down to the ankle, which will produce an added benefit to the ankle, tendons and muscles.

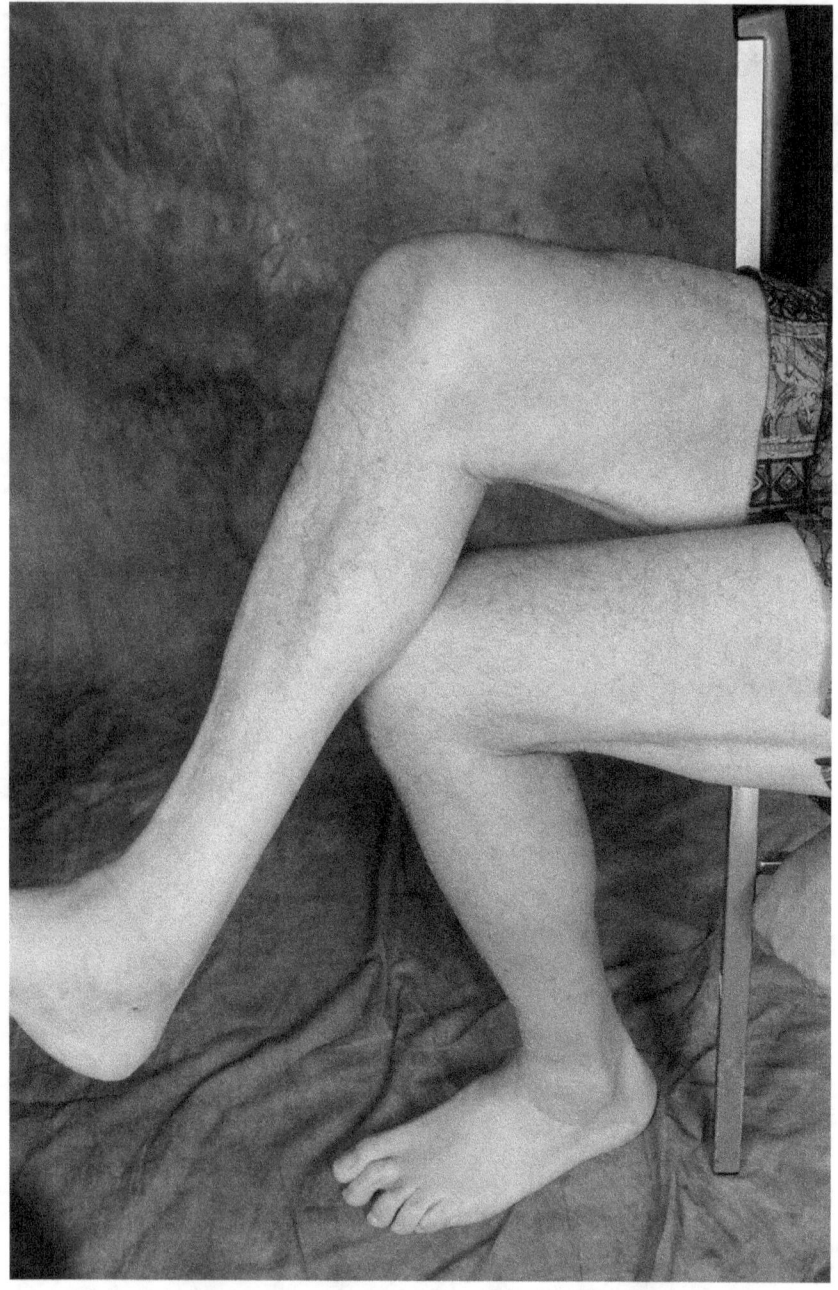

Figure 5: Calf to knee technique.

Another very useful technique is to flex the calves by doing toe raises. While standing, raise your body weight upon the tiptoe. You can do it with both feet, or you can double the strain on each calf by doing single-foot raises. A word of caution is if you have difficulty keeping your balance. You need to make sure you have a firm support that you can grab on to while doing the toe raises. Doing them in a doorway or next to a table would be a good method.

Sometimes I get a little lazy and do these calf flexes while sitting in a chair, but one must be careful not to push back too far, for fear of losing balance and breaking something - like your own bones.

When I first started to do toe raises, I couldn't do very many, especially the one-foot toe raises. Today I can do a hundred or more on both feet. In fifteen seconds, I can do twenty on one foot. Don't try to match this right away. Remember, it takes time. Start out slowly, using the thumb or knuckle massage. Do this once or twice a day building up to four or six times a day. Once the muscle is fully developed decrease the number to once or twice a day. If you begin to experience pain, stop the exercises until the next day. Pay special attention to your body when it becomes sore. You may have to take a day off to rest it. Sometimes I found myself working my body so hard I would have to stop and take a pain reliever to relax. This is not a good idea. Having to take pain relievers means that you are pushing your body too hard. Go easy at the start and build up gradually.

The secret to reversing the aging process is to work the muscles repetitively, six or more times a day. After the muscle has become fully developed decrease, the number of times.

These calf exercises will only take a few minutes a day. This is where you retirees have the advantage. Your time is your own. And you are the ones who are most concerned about aging, aren't you? You only have to massage each muscle for a short period of time, less than one minute per group. You can massage your whole body in less than ten minutes. It will depend on how long you want to spend on each muscle group. You may want to spend a longer amount of time (I have spent two hours flexing and massaging my body in the evening watching TV). It depends on what kind of workout you want to perform. You have to figure out how long and how often, you want to do this procedure. This depends on your own personal goal. Your muscle will become sore, just like when lifting weights. Start out slow and increase the workouts. You also have to figure out the amount of pressure you use, remember it's called deep massage. You must apply pressure to each muscle group.

CHAPTER III:
The Upper Leg

The upper leg, from the knee to the hip, contains four major muscle groups, and they are large, powerful ones. There are three muscle groups on the front of the thigh, and one group on the rear. These latter muscles are referred to as the hamstring muscles. There are individual sets of muscles within each group. I will refer to these sets by their location: the middle, side, and back groups.

Massaging the upper leg begins by extending your leg straight out in front of you. Begin massaging the middle and side groups at the front of the upper leg. You should be able to identify each set easily. Using the fist method (form a fist), massage each set of muscles with your knuckles. Figure 6 illustrates how you use the knuckles to massage the inside of leg. Message the middle and outside of leg using the same method.

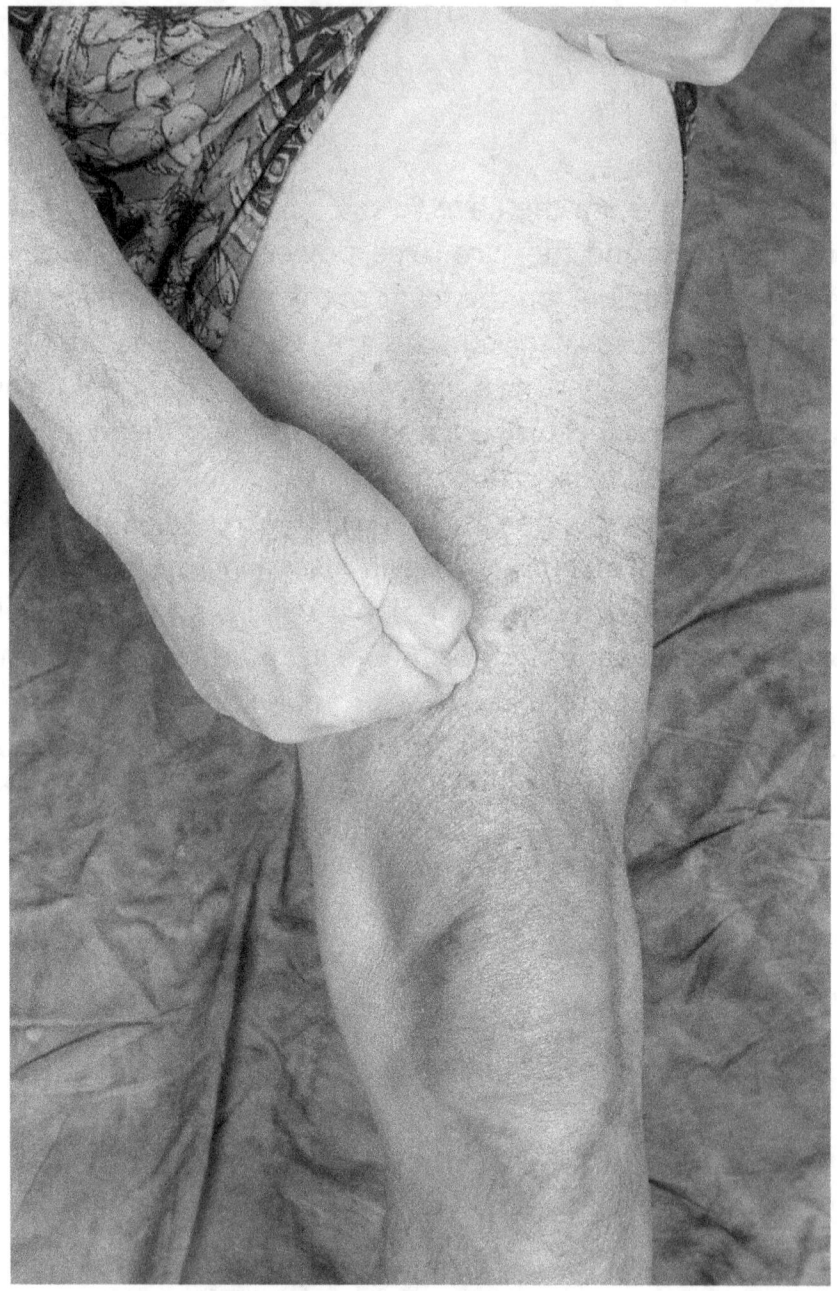

Figure 6: Knuckle technique.

There are as many options to massaging the upper leg as your imagination will allow. I have found it a useful technique to use my elbows in place of the knuckles. The elbow can be used to massage the top and inner muscle groups, as shown in Figures 7.

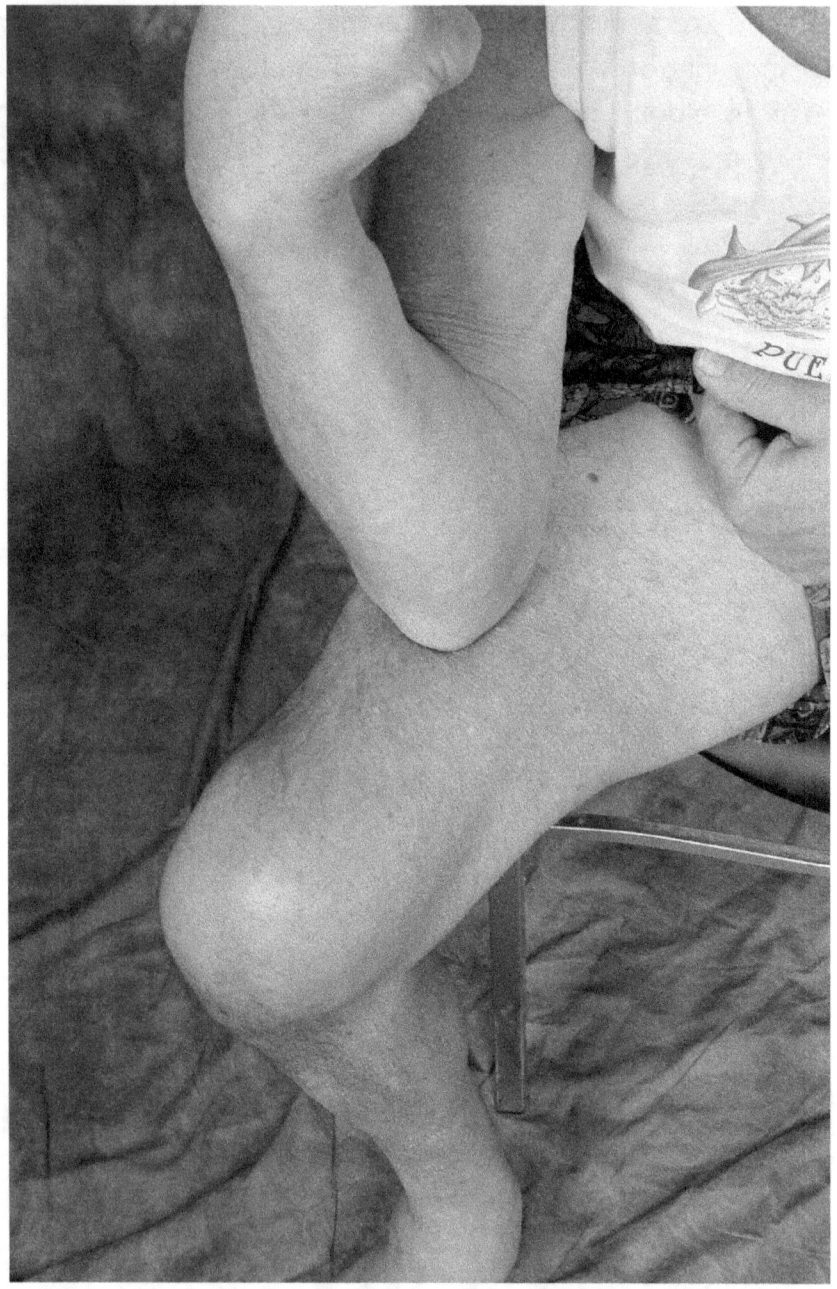

Figure 7: Elbow technique.

This method not only achieves the desired muscle massage, but also gives the arm and shoulder an extra workout.

Another technique involves the use of a massage stick, as illustrated in Figures 8.

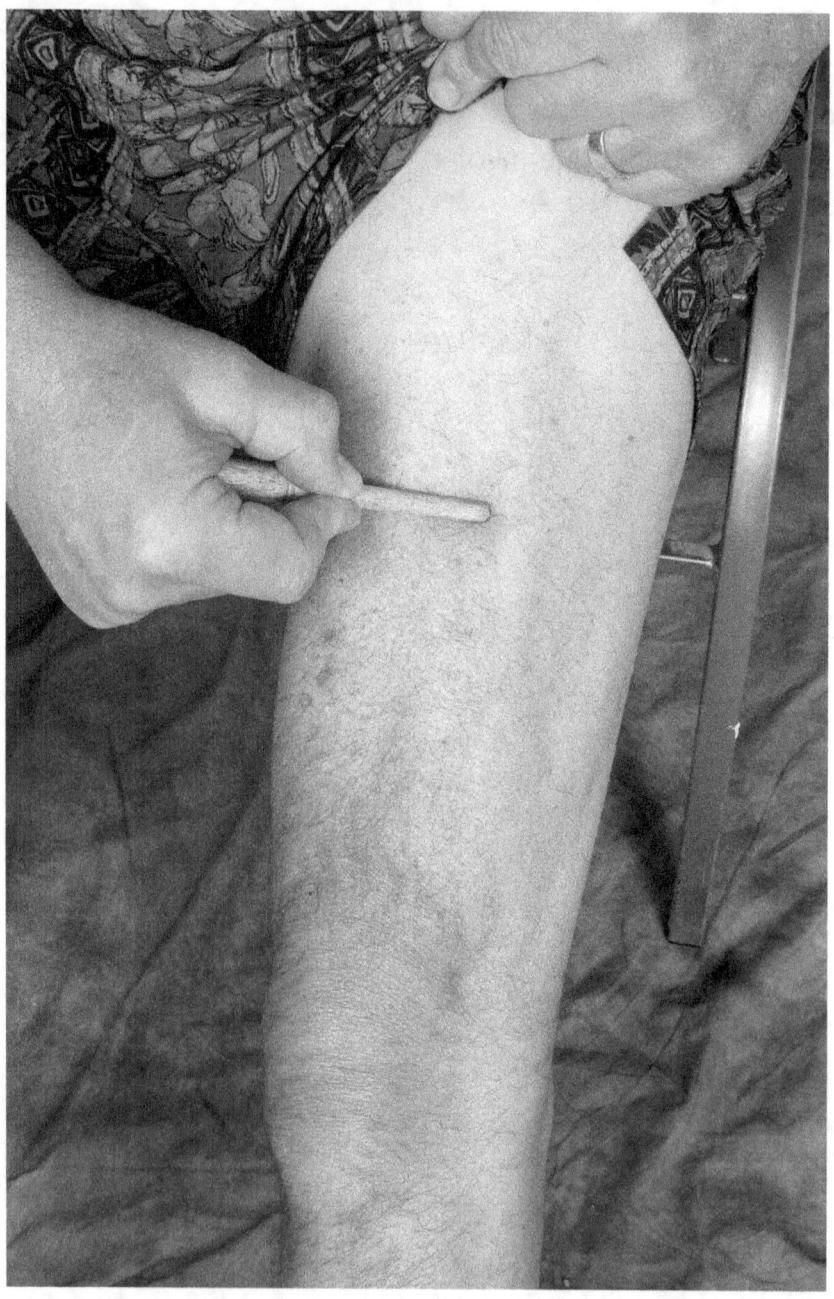

Figure 8

Massaging the back of the leg requires a different method. I found it best to cup the hand and use the fingers to massage up and down the leg. Alternatively, the massage stick - or your "rock buddy", as mentioned previously in Chapter II - can be used to massage the back of leg.

You should start out massaging your body twice a day, at the beginning and your goal is to massage the body six times a day. Once your muscle mass researches the 50% mark, after about four years. You should reduce the massaging to once or twice a day and concentrate more on flexing throughout the day. Your muscles will become sore, take a break, but don't give up. At times you may find it helpful to use a pain reliever such as Ibuprofen or Advil to relax the muscle. You should seek advice from your doctor if the pain persists. Your pain might be caused by something else. As with all exercise regimens you should seek advice from your physician first.

There is no need to strip down for these massage sessions. You can massage your muscles even when fully clothed. I frequently massage myself while I'm playing card, watching TV or just about any other activity where I'm relaxing. When you get used to a routine, you can massage at any time throughout the day. To reverse the normal aging process; It is important that you stimulate your muscles throughout the day. Occasional massage sessions are not enough. It is repetitious stimulation that pays off.

In addition to the massaging exercises we have been discussing, it is beneficial to flex the muscles too. My technique for flexing the upper leg is to sit with the ankle of one leg resting across the knee of the other leg. (Please note that those who have hip problems may not be able to do this). Press down on the knee with your ankle. You will feel the calf and outer thigh muscles stretching and tightening as you do this. Continue flexing the leg in this manner as long as you can, remember to start out slowly and gradually increase the tempo. The technique is illustrated in Figure 9.

Sit in chair, place feet out in front of chair on the floor lean back in chair, picking front legs of chair off the floor this will place pressure on upper leg, raise and lower legs of chair from floor, do as many as you can in one minute and do three sets,(fig. 10).

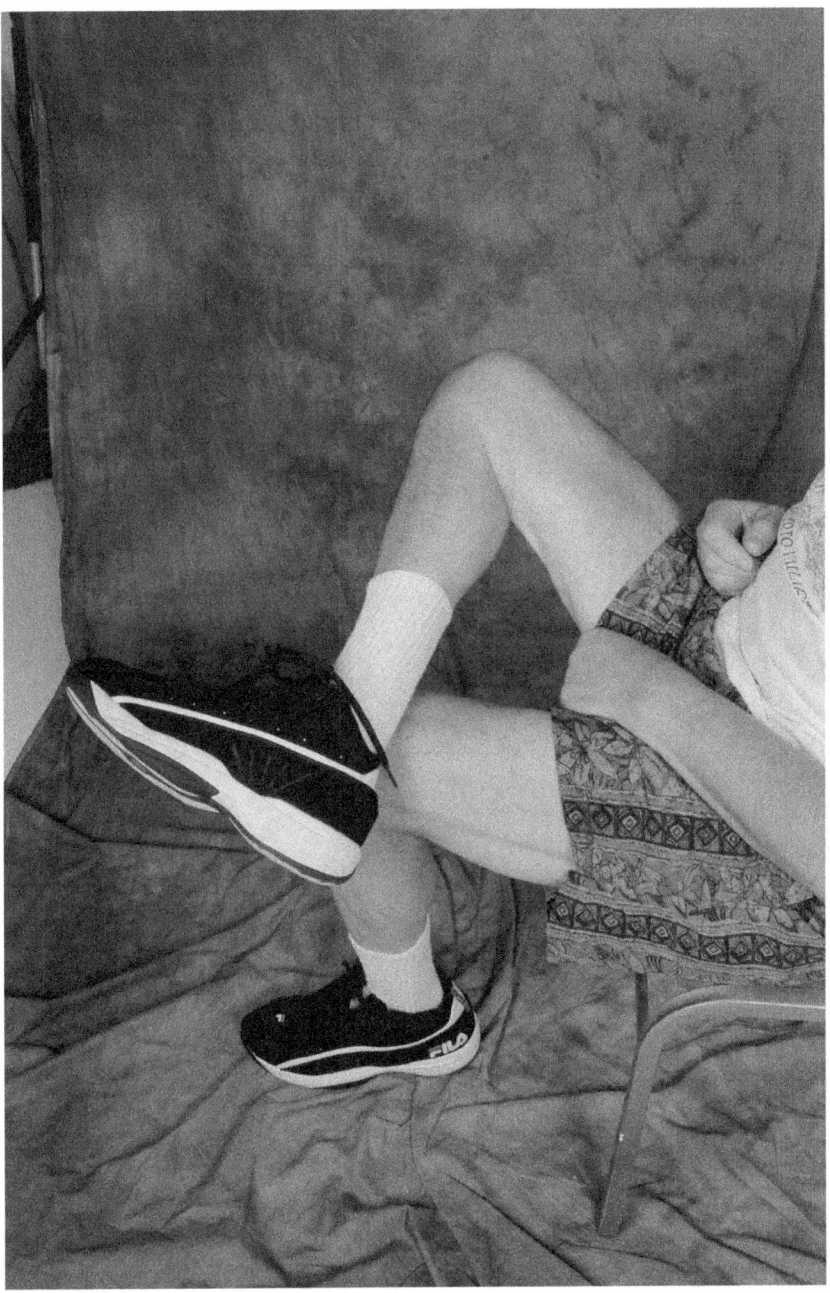

Figure 9

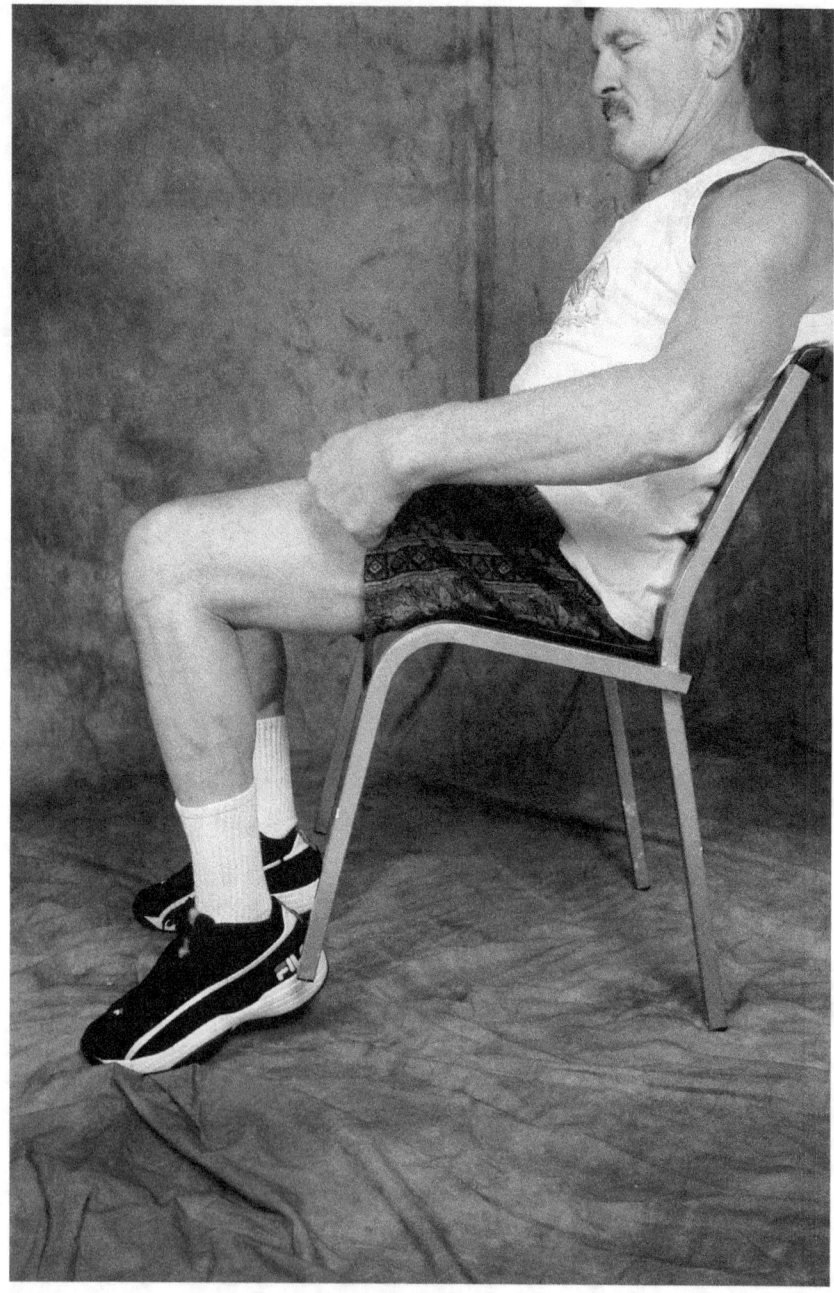

Figure 10

Remember to start out slowly and ease into it, gradually increasing the repetitions. When I first started I couldn't do very many repetitions.

At the age of sixty, before I started my flexing and massaging routines, I was having terrible problems. I liked to go fishing along the river. But getting down the fifteen-foot river bank was extremely difficult. I would have to sit down and slide down the bank, keeping a tight grip on my fishing gear all the while. At the end of my day I had to crawl back up the bank on my knees, grabbing branches to pull myself up. After a day of fishing I would hobble back to my car, unable to walk on the flat of my feet. I was forced to walk on the outside of my feet due to the pain. Today, just four years later, I laugh at these images.

Every year I would accompany my wife to a local Sewing Exposition. Last year I found it necessary to sit down frequently to rest my feet and legs. This year was a totally different story. I was able to walk through the entire grounds of the Sewing Expo. I was on my feet continuously for three hours. All the while I was flexing, stretching, and massaging my arm and thigh muscles. Over the course of three hours, I had no pain or discomfort. I did not require downtime to rest because I had no foot pains.

Here is another great leg flexing exercise: While standing upright, tense your leg muscles, concentrating on the calves and thighs. Hold this position for twenty seconds. Gradually increase the duration and number of flexes. You can do these flexing exercises throughout the day. It is important to stimulate the leg muscles daily to help reverse the aging process.

CHAPTER IV:
Hand Massage

It is probably not an exaggeration to say that for most people the hands and arms are the most used parts of their bodies. Whether from spending long periods of time at a computer, playing a sport, or just doing day-to-day chores. So it should be no surprise when I tell you that massaging the hands and forearms will be of immeasurable benefit to practically everyone.

Many of you may have discovered that at the age of sixty the joints of our hands, and indeed many other parts of your body, may be developing arthritis. Just as mine did. Arthritis is the swelling of the joints, which is an unfortunate accompaniment of aging for many of us. Additionally, the complexity of the hands, coupled with the strain we are forced to subject them to over a lifetime, makes them highly susceptible to tendon and bone damage. I will discuss both of these problems in this and the following chapters.

Sports activities also contribute seriously to tendon and joint problems. Golfers and baseball players, for example, are especially vulnerable to the severe shocks transmitted from the club head or the bat directly into the joints and tendons of the hands, wrists, and arm joints. This can cause serious harm that often doesn't become noticeable until later in life. In my own case, I love golf. But the constant hitting of the golf ball at the driving range or on the course caused serious pains and swelling to develop.

Tendonitis is another source of pain in the hands, wrists, and elbow joints. Strong or repetitive movement, such as those occurring in golf, tennis, baseball, etc., can create excessive friction between the surface of a tendon and the bones over which it is stretched. The condition known as tennis elbow is a familiar example.

Another source of tendon problems is calcification of the joints. When calcium spurs build up on a bone, and a tendon has to stretch across it, the tendon may become inflamed and sometimes frayed, causing severe pain whenever the joint is moved.

To obtain maximum benefit from hand massage, you should massage each finger for thirty seconds or more. Each finger should be massaged all the way from the base to the tip. Two methods are required. First, you should use small circular massage motions starting at the base of the finger and work gradually toward the tip. Secondly, use long, smooth strokes, again from the base to tip. The long massage stroke should be repeated on the upper (back side) and bottom (palm side) of each finger, as well as along the sides. Pay special attention to the large knuckles of each finger by using circular massaging motions.

Now massage the palm of the hand, the base of the thumb, and the back of the hand using the knuckle method described earlier.

To massage the palm, you place the thumb of one hand on the palm of the opposite hand and apply pressure, holding the pressure for two or three seconds. Move the thumb over the surface of the palm as you continue to apply pressure. Switch hands and repeat the procedure on your other hand.

If you are tired of using your thumb to apply the pressure, try using the "rock buddy" I mentioned in Chapter I.

Another great hand exercise is to tense them in a series of alternate squeezing and stretching motions. Start by forming a fist and squeeze it as hard as possible for twenty seconds. Pretend you're Mohammed Ali getting ready to deliver a left or right jab. Then, relax your fist and open the hand to extend and spread the fingers out as far as possible. Hold the hand open in this manner for an additional twenty seconds.

Stretching the fingers is beneficial. Stretch them by pushing back at the top of the fingers with your other hand, as far as is comfortable. This will stretch all of your hand joints: fingers, hand, and wrist.

CHAPTER V:

Forearms

The techniques for massaging and flexing the arm are almost
the same as those used on the legs. With a little practice,
you will find arm massage just as rewarding. Arm massage
has beneficial effects not only for the arms, but also for the
hands and shoulders. The reasons for this are not that obvi-
ous, but are well worth noting. Any movement of massaging
or flexing one arm involves the use of the opposite hand, arm,
and shoulder. So you get double the benefit from this set of
treatments.

Not surprisingly, tension in your arms can cause aches
and pains in your shoulder and neck. For all of these parts
are connected to one another. As the song says, "arm bone's
connected to the shoulder bone", etc.

Because of the relative strength of the arm and shoulder
muscles, you will find that strong movements are required to
unlock tension in these muscles and tendons.

The bones of the arm have a similar arrangement to those
of the leg, on a smaller scale. The upper arm bone, or humerus, is joined to the lower arm bones, the ulna and radius,
at the elbow joint.

To massage the forearm muscle, you use the fist method,
going up and down the muscle between the two bones. Use
deep massage to stimulate the muscle (a process of breaking
down the muscle fiber so the muscle will grow).

You can also use a massage stick covering the same area.
As shown in figures 11 and 12.

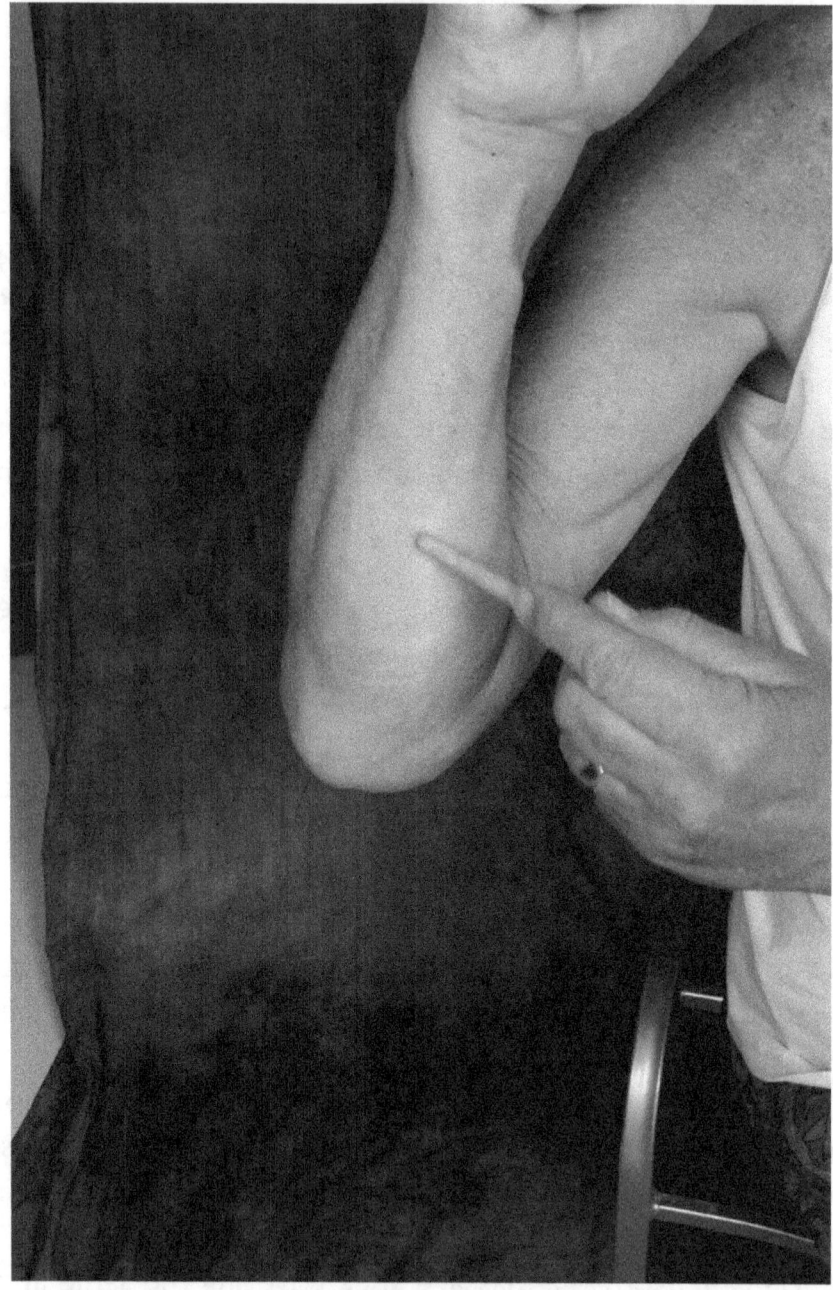

Figure 11

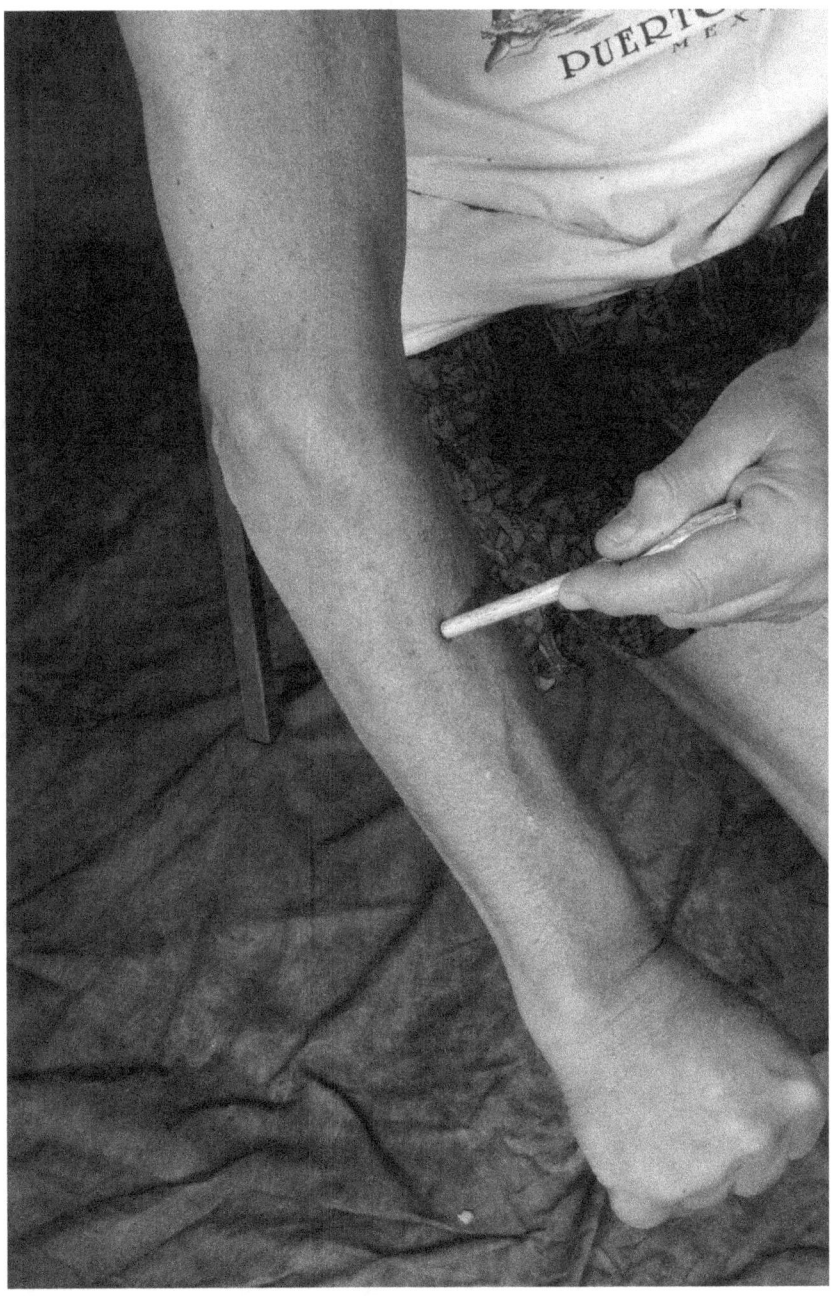

Figure 12

You can also stroke one forearm with the other forearm, slowly rotating the top forearm as you stroke from the elbow to the wrist of your other arm. This stroke massages both arms simultaneously and is very effective.

When I first started to deep massage my forearms, they became sore and tender due to breaking down and stimulation of the muscles. I found that at night I had to keep my arms straight so they wouldn't lose circulation and go to sleep. I started out using very hard and vigorous massaging to maximize the result. You may want to start out slower and gradually build up to the vigorous pace that I used. This only seemed to happen with my deltoids and forearms.

CHAPTER VI:

Upper Arms

The main muscles in the upper arm are the deltoids, the biceps, and the triceps. The deltoids are the large bands of muscle that move the arms across your chest. They are attached to the collar bone at the upper end and the humerus, or upper arm bone, at the other. The biceps are on the front part of the upper arm, and are used to flex the arms and do the arm-curl exercises. The triceps are at the back of the arm and are used to straighten the arm. These big muscles all respond well to deep, firm massage.

To massage the bicep, use the fist method and massage each side and top of bicep. Continue the bicep massage by cupping the bicep with the opposite hand. Using the thumb, push inward, applying pressure to massage the inner side of the bicep. Then, using your fingers, push down to massage the top of the bicep. Move the fingers to the outside of the bicep to massage the outer part, pushing in firmly with the fingers. Repeat the same methods on other arm. You can also use a massage stick (figures 13 and 14).

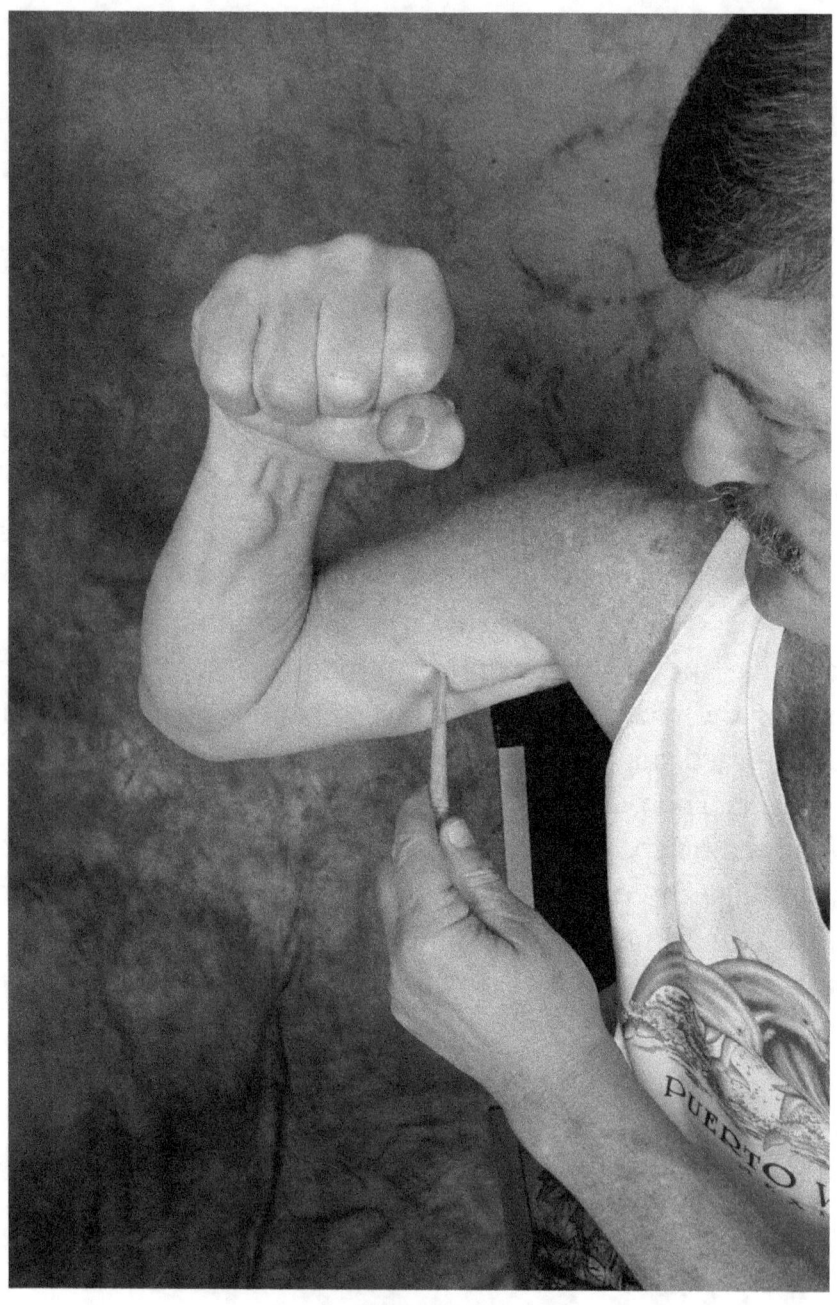

Figure 13

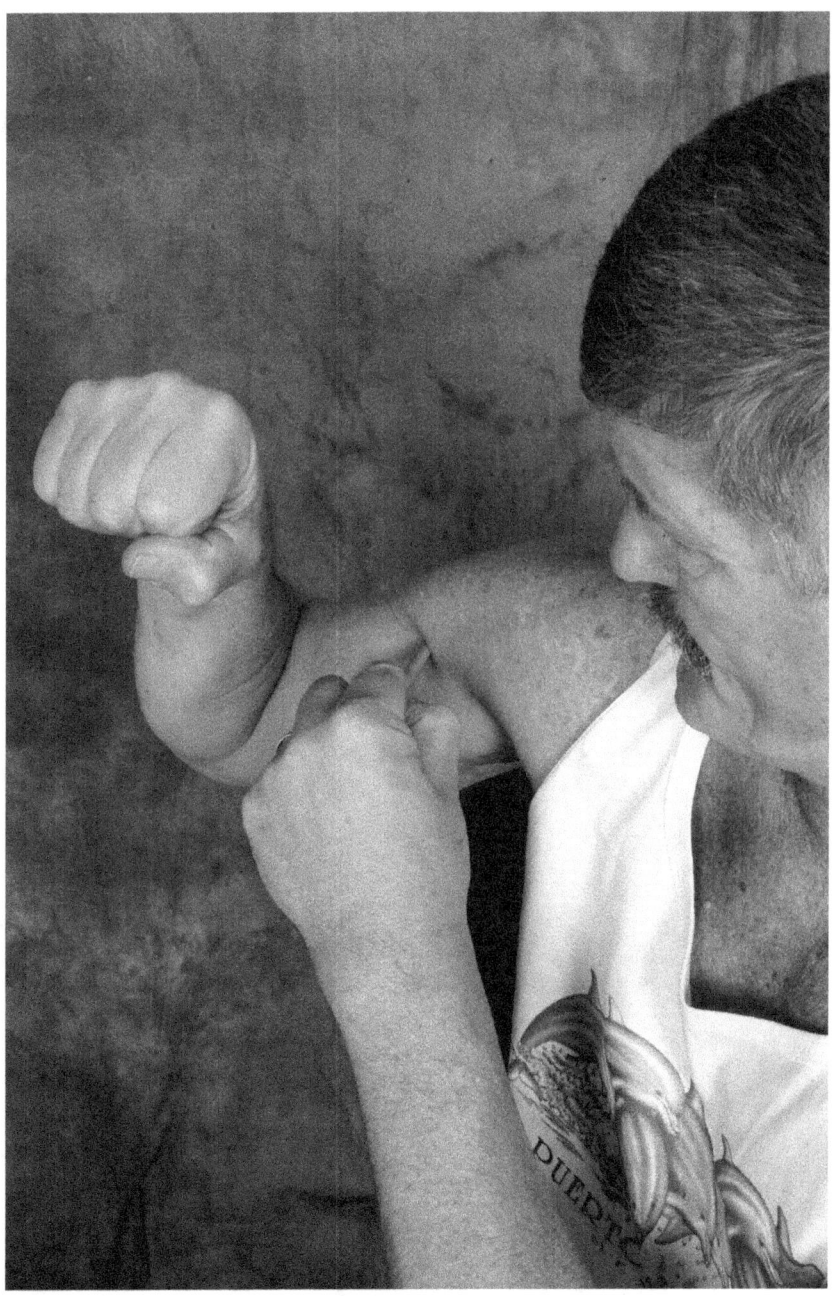

Figure 14

To massage the triceps, you hold the arm straight down, cup the muscle in your hand, and massage it with your fingertips, squeezing the muscle all the way up and down its length and from side to side. You may also use the fist method or the massage stick. Go up and down the length of the triceps, massaging the entire muscle to stimulate growth.   Repeat these procedures on other arm, figure 15.

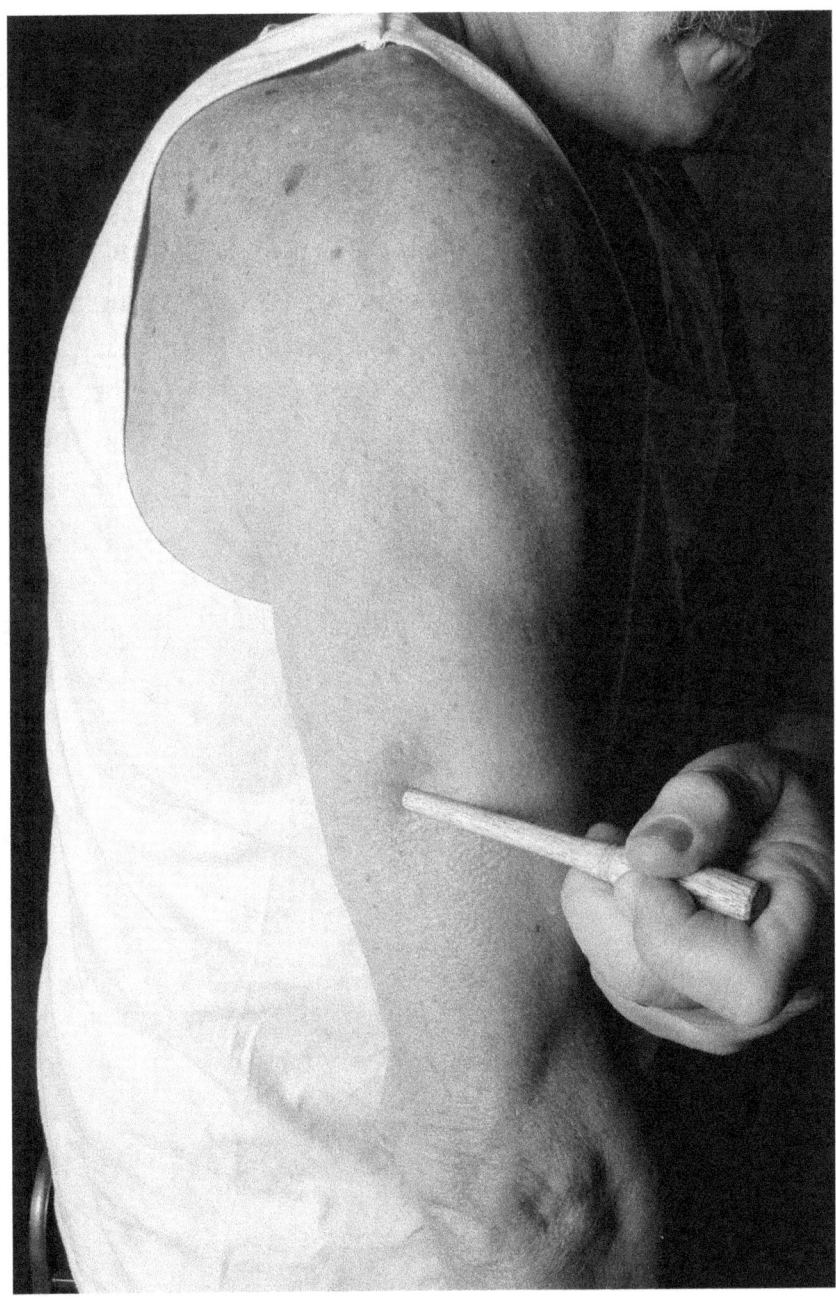

Figure 15

Now for the big deltoid muscles: cup the muscle with your thumb on the side of the collar bone, and use your fingers to massage each muscle area. Push down with the fingers, going up and down its length and from side to side, just as with the other arm muscles. You may also use the fist, or massage stick, methods by going up and down the length of the muscles, as shown in Figure 16. Be careful not to over-stimulate the deltoid muscles, as they can become painful, and will bother you at night. It is always best to start out slowly and gradually work up to the more energetic massaging. The muscle responds and will grow quickly.

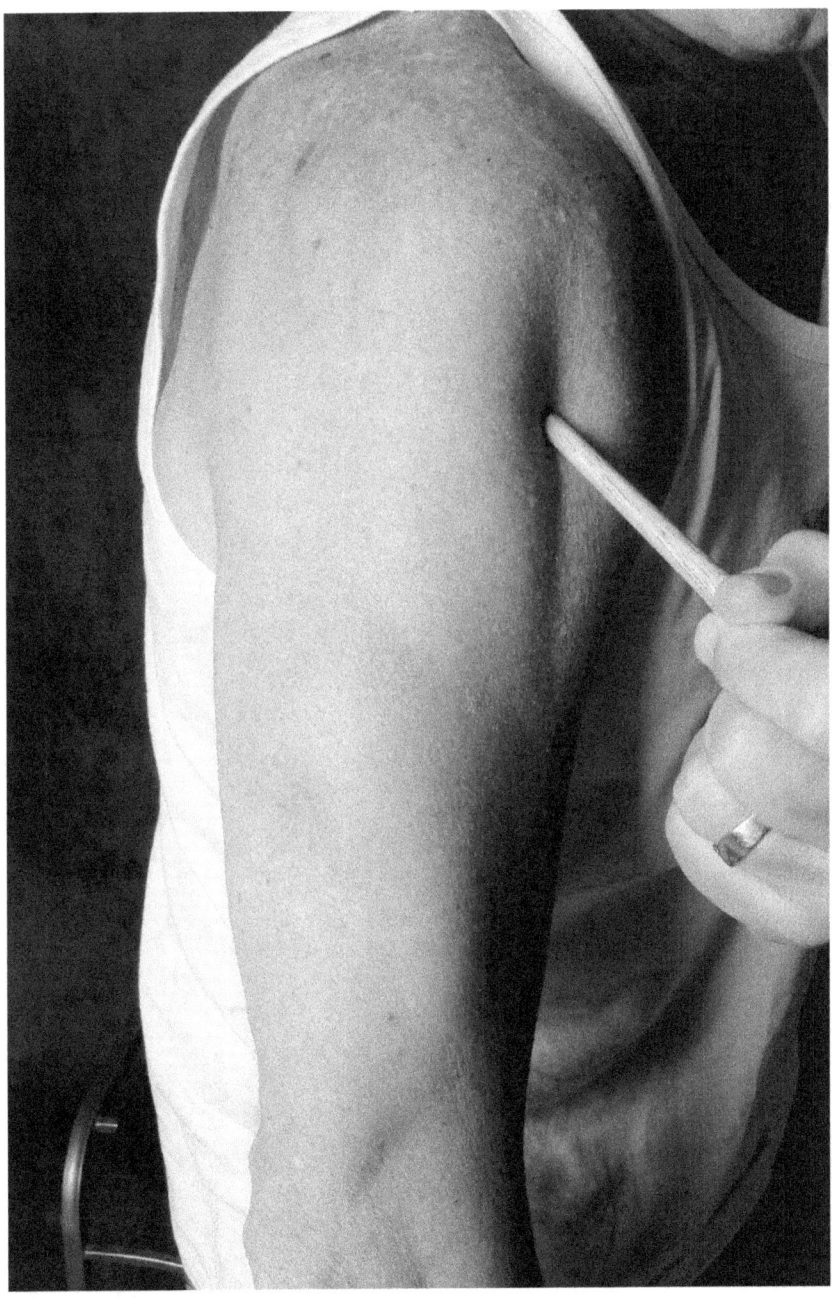

Figure 16

Let us turn now to flexing of the forearm and biceps. To flex these muscles, simply bend your arm and rotate the fist to the left and right, as in Figure 17.

The triceps and deltoids are flexed with the arm pointed straight down. Turn the fist in and out, as shown Figure 18.

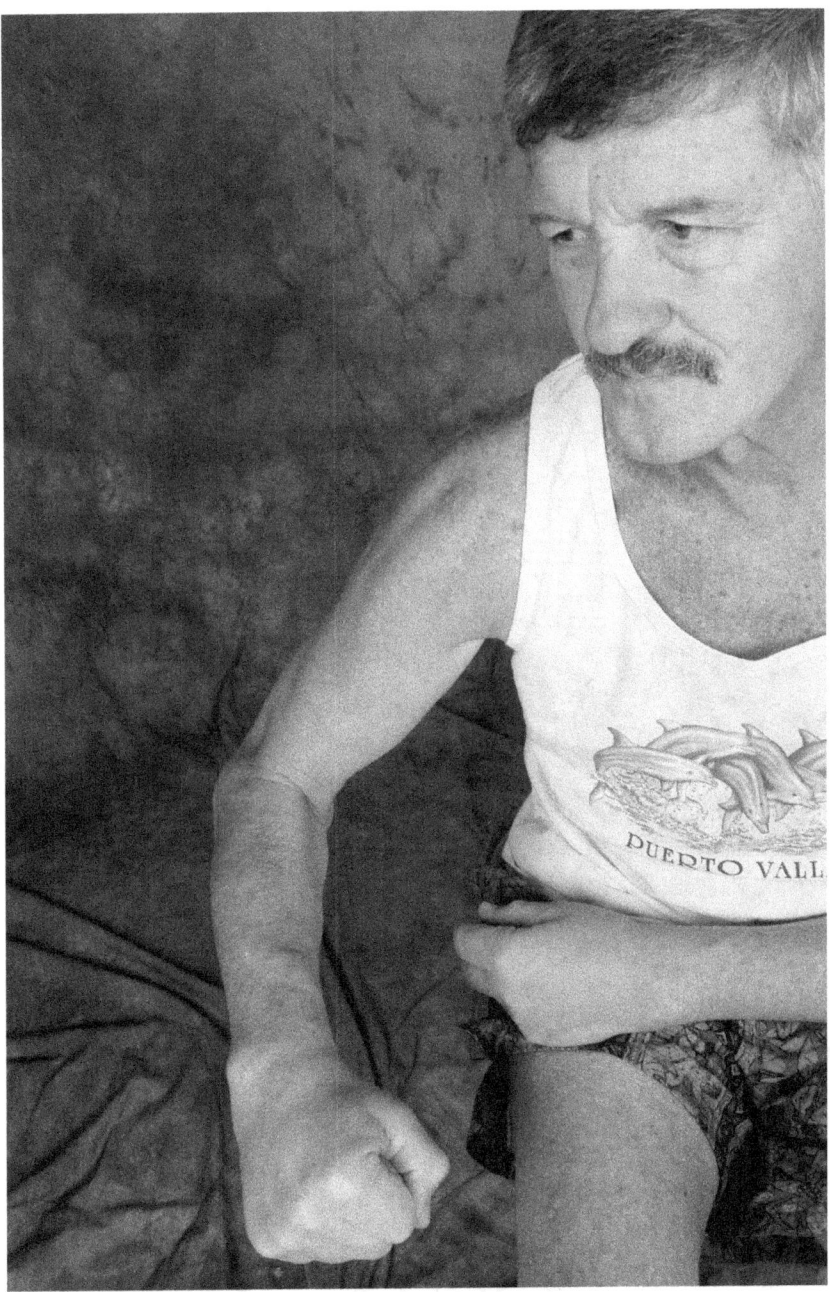

Figure 17

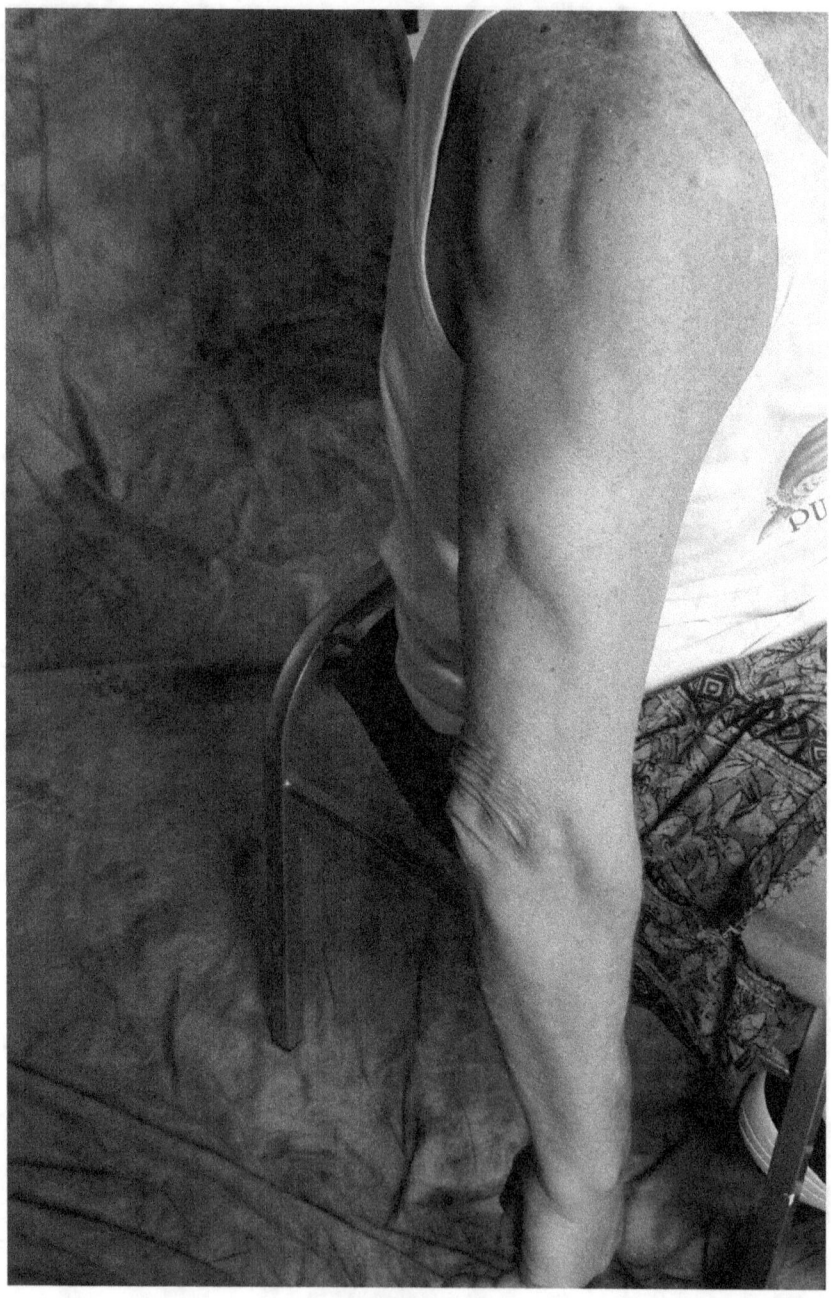

Figure 18

Here are a couple of very good exercises you can perform while sitting in an armchair. Bend your arms, place the elbows on the inside of the chair-arms and push out with your elbows against the side of the chair-arms. Then place your elbows on outside of the chair-arms and pull your elbows inward. These are very good exercises for the upper arms, and can be done while you are otherwise relaxing.

You can massage these areas while wearing street clothing. You just massage through the clothing. This way you can continue to massage throughout the day, taking just a few minutes at a time. It is important to keep the muscles stimulated throughout the day.

When you first start to stimulate your arms with deep massage, you will find that it produces the same effect as lifting weights: The arms will become sore. This means that your muscles are growing and you are reversing your aging process. You are becoming younger, more vigorous, as you age. Start out gradually and remember to talk to your physician before starting into this program.

When I first started to massage my muscles (examples triceps). There was a space between the muscles, like a hole between the sets of muscles. This was an example of the muscles turning into fat tissues and fiber. The muscles were turning into flab, which is a part of the aging process. Now the muscle is a solid mass of muscles which shows a reversal of the aging process.

CHAPTER VII:
Neck, Shoulder And Chest

Most people suffer from tension and pain in their necks and shoulder at some time in their lives. Consider the job that the neck and shoulders have to do. Bad posture, stress, lifting heavy objects, performing different sports activities, all conspire to make the problem worse. But even the sheer weight of your head can often cause your neck and shoulders to ache. You can ease the pain and stress by developing the strength and size of these muscles, through flexing and massaging. This simple self-massage exercise gets right to the core of the tension and eases it. You can try it almost anywhere and at any time. Try to focus on the areas that feel most tense, and work slowly, deeply and methodically.

Stroke your hands up and down the back of your neck to warm the muscle in the area. Place fingers of both hands at the back of neck on either side of the spinal column. Use the fingers and thumb pads of both your hands to squeeze and make deep pressure all around the back of the neck, making sure that you do not apply pressure to the spinal column itself. Cup the back of the neck, placing the thumb on the left side of the neck and fingers on the right side. Squeeze and make deep pressure on the back of neck muscles with the thumb and fingers. Reverse hand and do process again on other side of neck.

Take your left index finger placing it on the right side of your neck between the neck muscle and your Adam's apple. Apply pressure with finger rubbing up and down your neck, making sure that you do not apply pressure to the Adam's apple. Repeat massage on left side of neck (using your left hand). This should stimulate the muscles in the neck, making the neck look younger, figure 19.

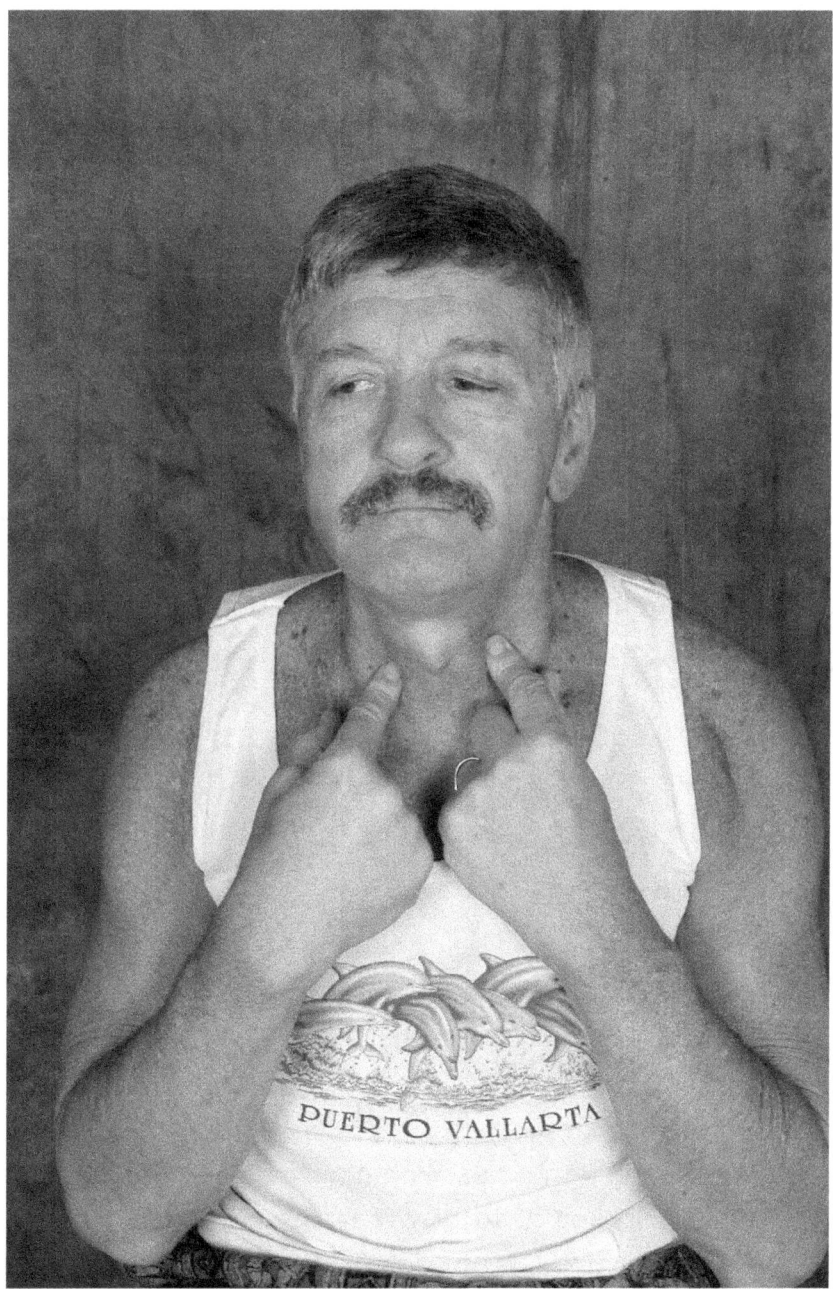

Figure 19

Place your left hand on your right shoulder and squeeze the muscle. Hold the squeeze and slowly rotate your shoulder backward. A grinding noise indicates that the muscles are tense and should be freed up. Repeat with the right hand on the left shoulder.

With your finger or fist, stroke firmly from the center of your chest outward, applying deep pressure between your chest towards your armpit. When your fingers reach the outer edges of your chest, return to the center and repeat the movement. Feel for tense spots and concentrate on these as you work over the chest, example figure 20.

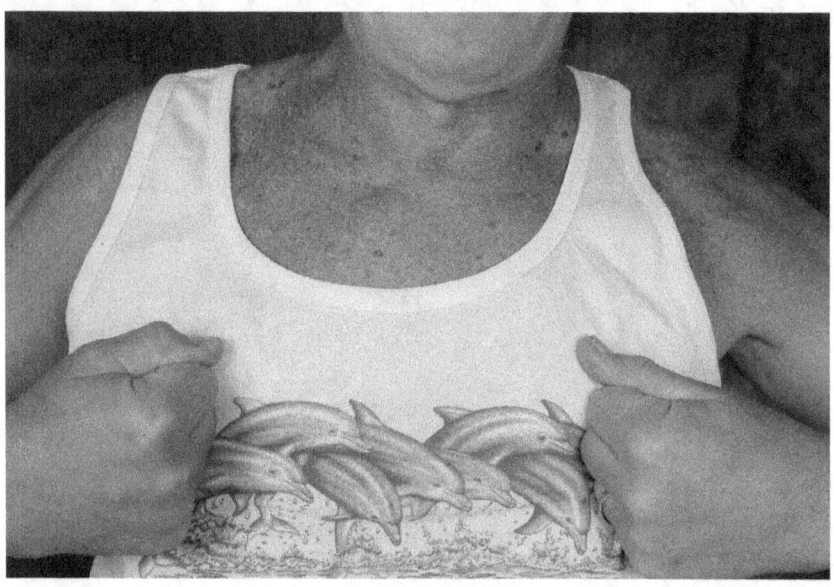

Figure 20

Flexing the neck muscles. Form a fist. Place the fist under your chin; push your head down against your fist, figure 21. This will put pressure on the back of your neck muscles. Place your fist on the right side of your chin; push your head against your fist, figure 22. This will put pressure on the left side of your neck muscles. Repeat exercise to other side.

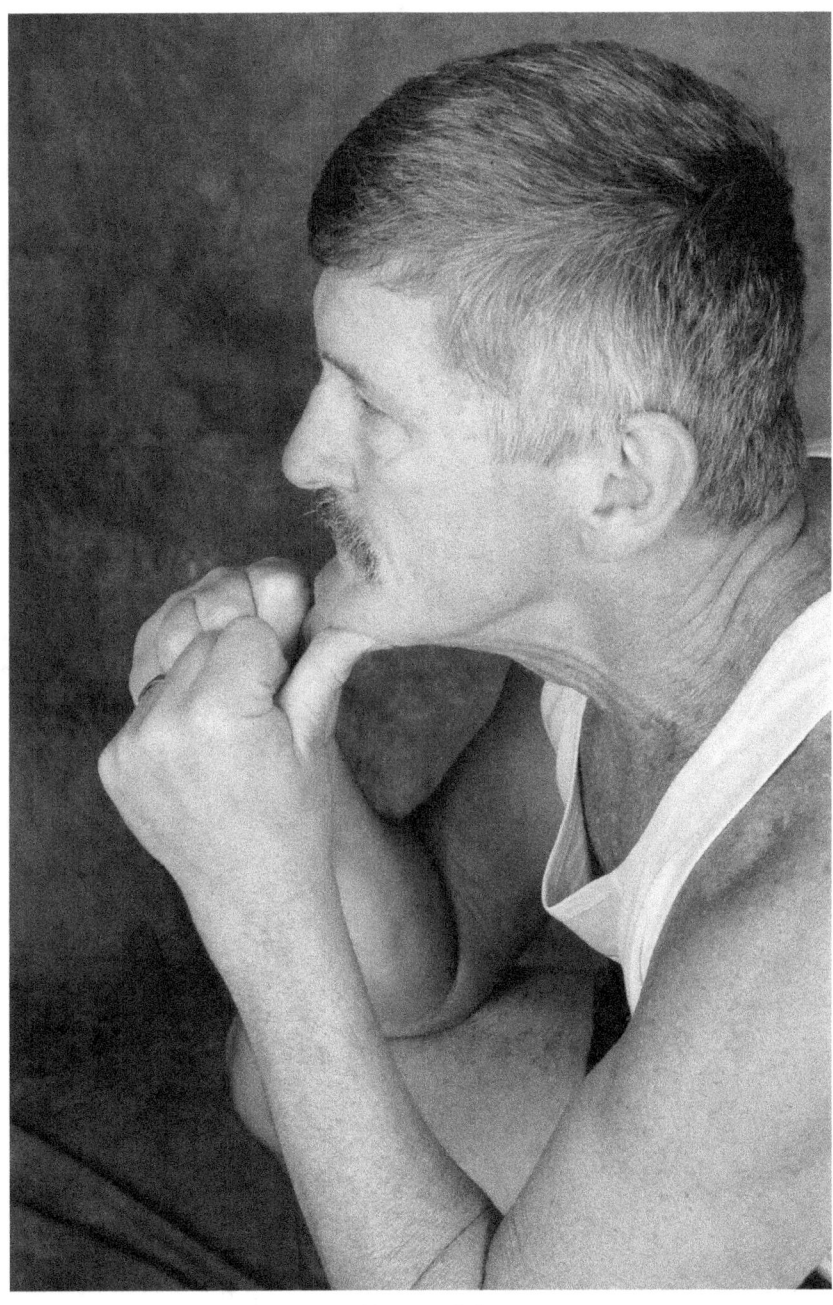

Figure 21

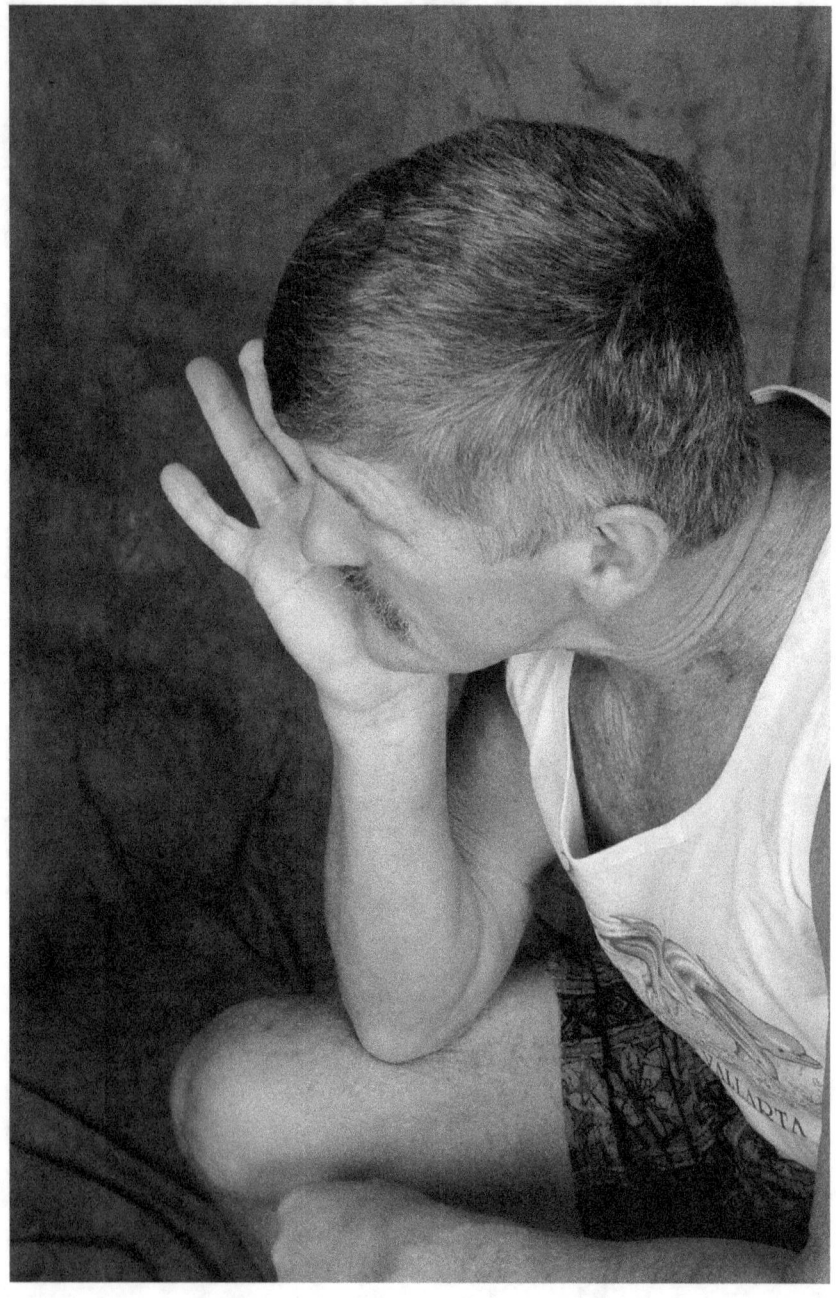

Figure 22

Make a series of thumb pressures on the muscles between the ribs. Start in the middle and work up and down the rib cage. You also can use the fist method, figure 23. Pressure in this area can be painful, so be guided by the pain when deciding on the amount of pressure you apply.

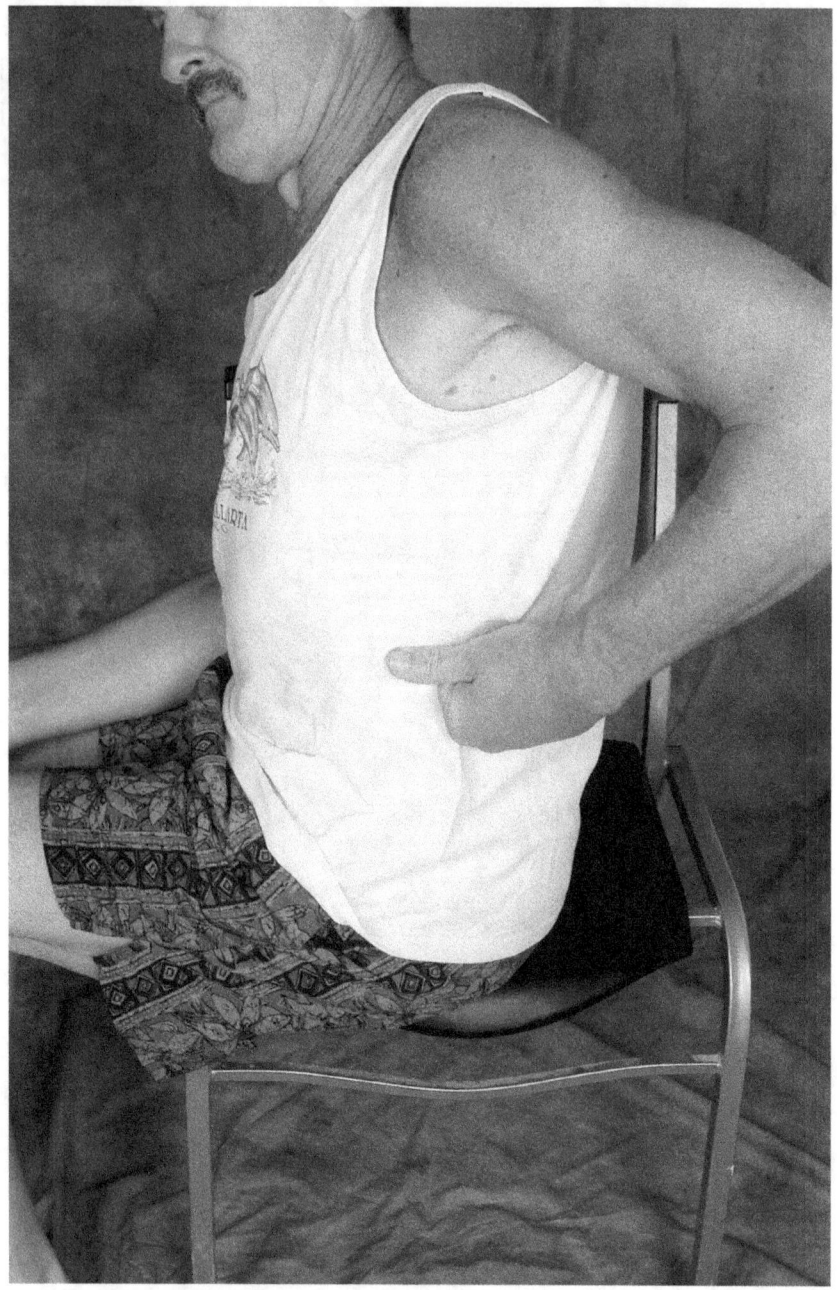

Figure 23

The muscle in front of the armpit is called the pectoral. If the muscle became soft and flabby, it has turned into fat tissue and fiber. Pick up and squeeze the muscle, on the right side with your left hand. Squeeze from the armpit to the nipple. Repeat this procedure on the left side. Over a period of time this muscle will become firm and muscular.

Flexing the shoulder and chest muscles. Sit in a chair. Place your elbows on your thighs. Clasp your hands together; between your knees and flex (tighten) your shoulder and chest muscles. This will put pressure on these muscles. Hold flex for twenty seconds. Repeat this exercise three times.

CHAPTER VIII:
Back, Abdomen And Buttocks

Abdomen - It's natural to rub your abdomen when you have a stomach ache. Any form of abdominal massage, however basic, is extremely comforting. You can massage your abdomen while sitting up. Always use a clockwise motion when massaging the abdomen since this follows the working of the intestine. This can help relax the abdomen, which, in-turn, can aid digestion.

Stroke one hand after the other around your abdomen in a clockwise direction, lifting one hand over the other in a continuous flow. Increase the size of the circle to cover the whole area. Then gradually make it smaller again.

Apply circular pressure all around the abdomen. Use one hand on top of the other, or the palm of just one hand, depending on how much pressure you want to apply to stimulate the muscles.

Lower back - You can massage your lower back by sitting forward in a chair. Start by vigorously rubbing the palms of both your hands up and down the small of your back, and from side-to-side, to warm the area and release any muscular tension.

For a stronger, deeper movement, make your hands into fists and press the thumb side of your hand into your sacrum, the lower part of your spine, figure 24. Then stroke your fists firmly up and down the area. Make deliberate, circular pressure with your fingertips and thumbs all around sacrum.

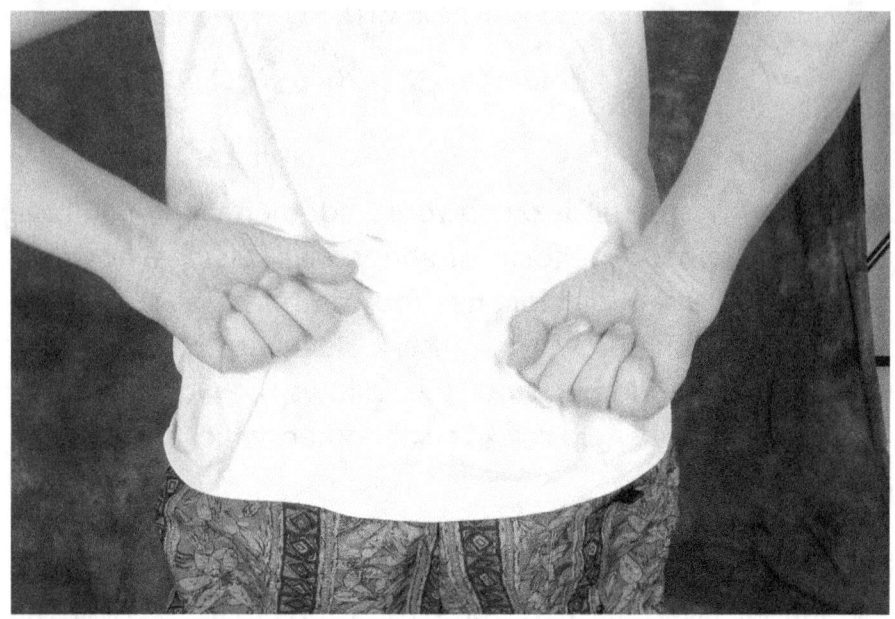

Figure 24

The buttock muscles are among the most powerful in the body. Lie on your right side. Place your left fist at the top of the buttock and stroke up and down and side-to-side covering the entire area. Also cup the buttock with the left hand applying pressure with your fingers covering the entire area. Repeat exercise to right side. When standing up massage up and down the entire buttock using the fist method, figure 25.

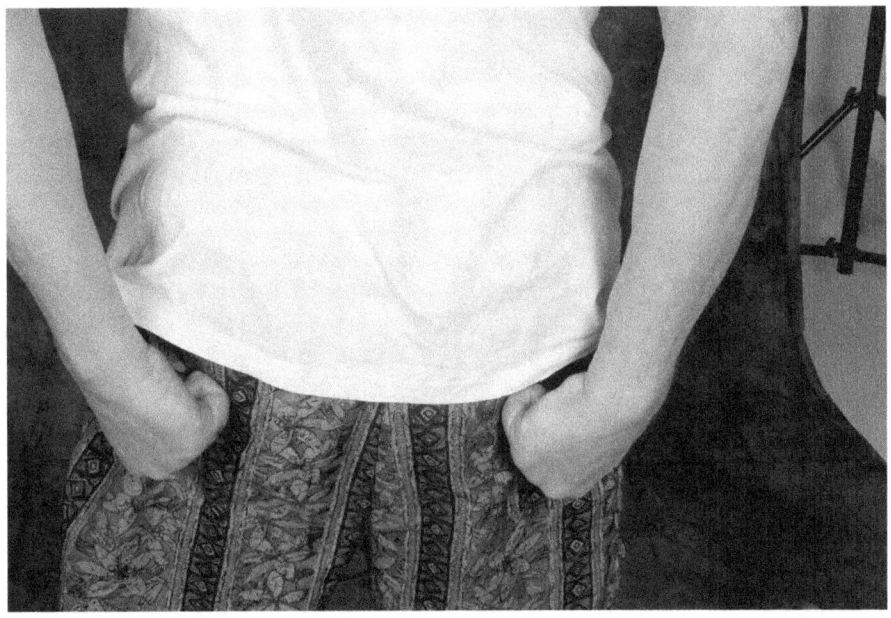

Figure 25

I have not found a way to massage the upper back by myself. But flexing the muscle has stimulated the muscle to grow replacing the fat tissue and fiber.

Flexing the stomach muscles, flex the muscle of the stomach. Flexing the buttock muscles tensing the back of the upper leg and buttock muscles.

CHAPTER IX:

Full Facial Massage

Full facial-This winter we went to a Christmas party for the grandchildren. I was sitting next to one of the distance relatives. We were sitting at the table alone, so I told her I was writing a book and we started talking about self-massage. I told her I was writing about facial massage. We talked about different techniques of facial massage. Then I asked her how old she was and of course she said "how old do you think I'm ". I replied "37 years", she replied "50". I was totally amazed she didn't have any wrinkles on her face. I asked her many questions about the techniques she used on her face. She started massaging her face at an early age in life around 30 years old. Remember the female body starts to age at 32 years old. I will share these techniques with you. The first thing I did when I got home was call my 35 year old daughter and shared this information with her.

So you are thinking I'm much older and what good is this information going to do for me. I started to massage my face at the age of 60. It was interesting that I would get up in the middle of the night and look in the mirror. My face would be all puffy and wrinkly. After massaging for a year, when I looked in the mirror in the middle of the night my faces would be smoother and would have less wrinkles. I was stimulating the muscle in the face turning the fat tissue and fiber back into muscle.

The face is especially well suited to self-massage. We instinctively stroke our foreheads when we have a headache and hold our forehead when concentrating. The face contains a huge number of nerve receptors. Therefore, a face massage can have profound effects all through the body, changing our mood, enhancing relaxation, and controlling pain.

Stroke your whole face with soft, molding hands. Then, with the fingers of both hands, stroke slowly and firmly from the center of your forehead out to your temples. Stroke under your cheekbones, from your nose to your ears. Then stroke from your mouth out toward the edges of your jaw.

Explore your face with circular finger pressures, moving your skin against the underlying muscles. Vary the size, depth, and direction of the circles; try flat, shallow circles and deep, penetrating spirals. Feel for any taut, overused muscles and pay particular attention to your jaw, since tension is often stored there.

Stroke your forehead with your right hand going from the top of the eyebrow to the top of the forehead only going straight up covering the whole forehead, figure 26. Then with the right hand stroke from the right temple to the left temple covering the whole forehead. Then with the right hand stroke across the forehead from the top of the eyebrow to the top of the forehead by always going up.

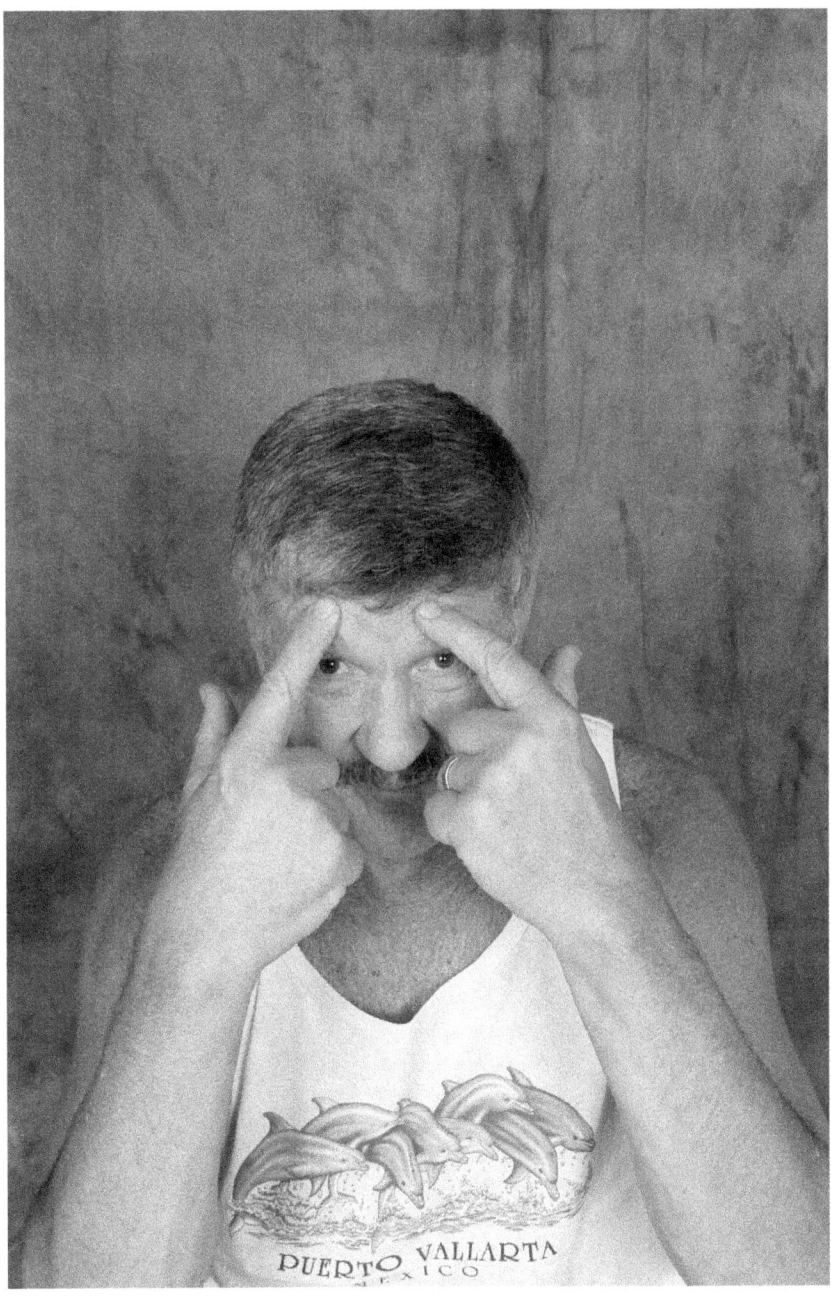

Figure 26

Gently stroke around your right eye with your right hand and your left eye with your left hand at the same time, figure 27. Then squeeze along each eyebrow from the bridge of your nose to your temples using your index fingers and thumbs.

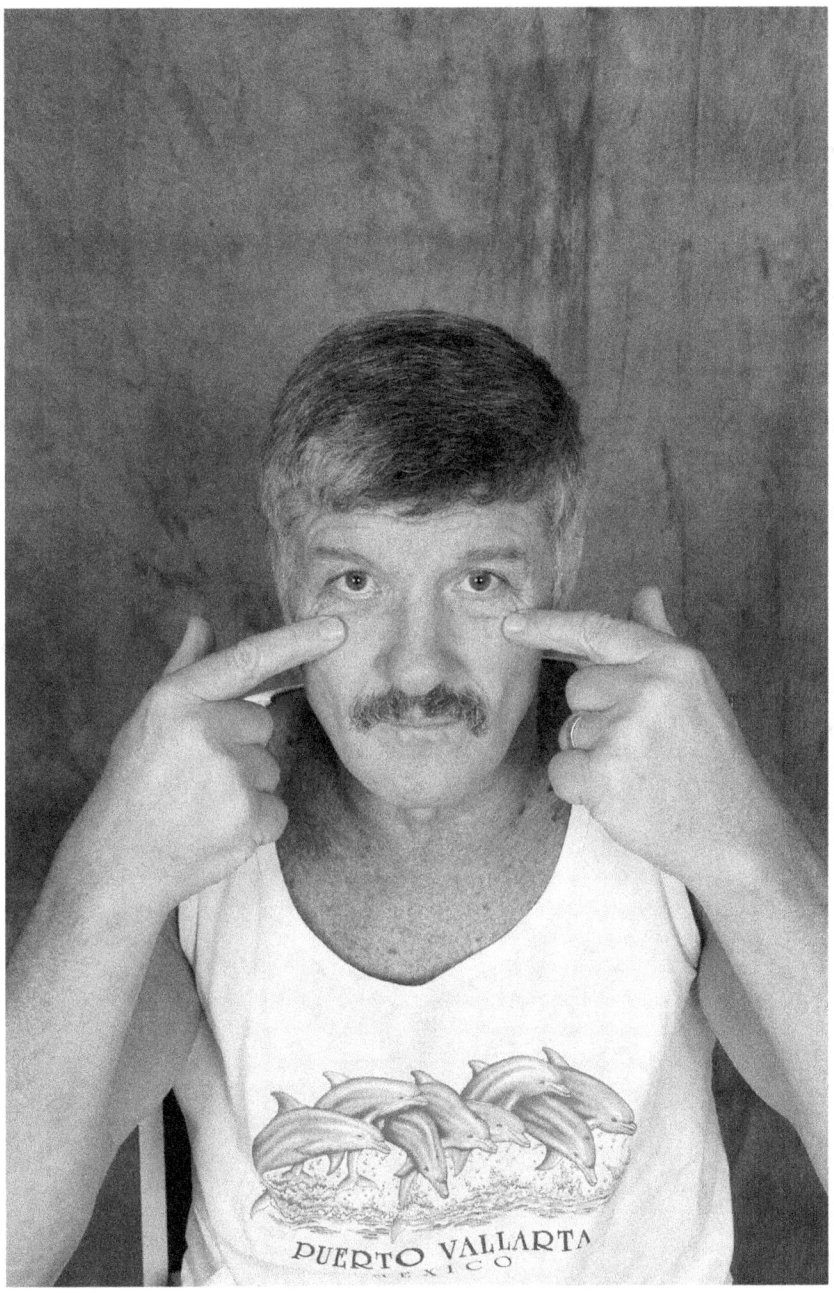

Figure 27

Stroke from the bridge of the nose down to the nostril, across the cheekbones and up to the temples. It helps to use the right hand on the right side and the left hand on the left side. Stroke under the cheekbones and also cover the whole cheek. Using the right and left thumb stroke out under the jaw to the ears. Pause for a moment with your palms resting over the ears, and then glide your thumbs back down under the chin. Stroke with your thumbs from the chin, around the mouth, to the nostrils. Continue stroking up the sides of the nose, pausing just below the eyes, then glide out under the cheekbones and up to the temples, and then return to the chin. Stroke with the index fingers from the base of the chin follow the jaw bone up to the temples, figure 28. Repeat each techniques several times and message twice a day.

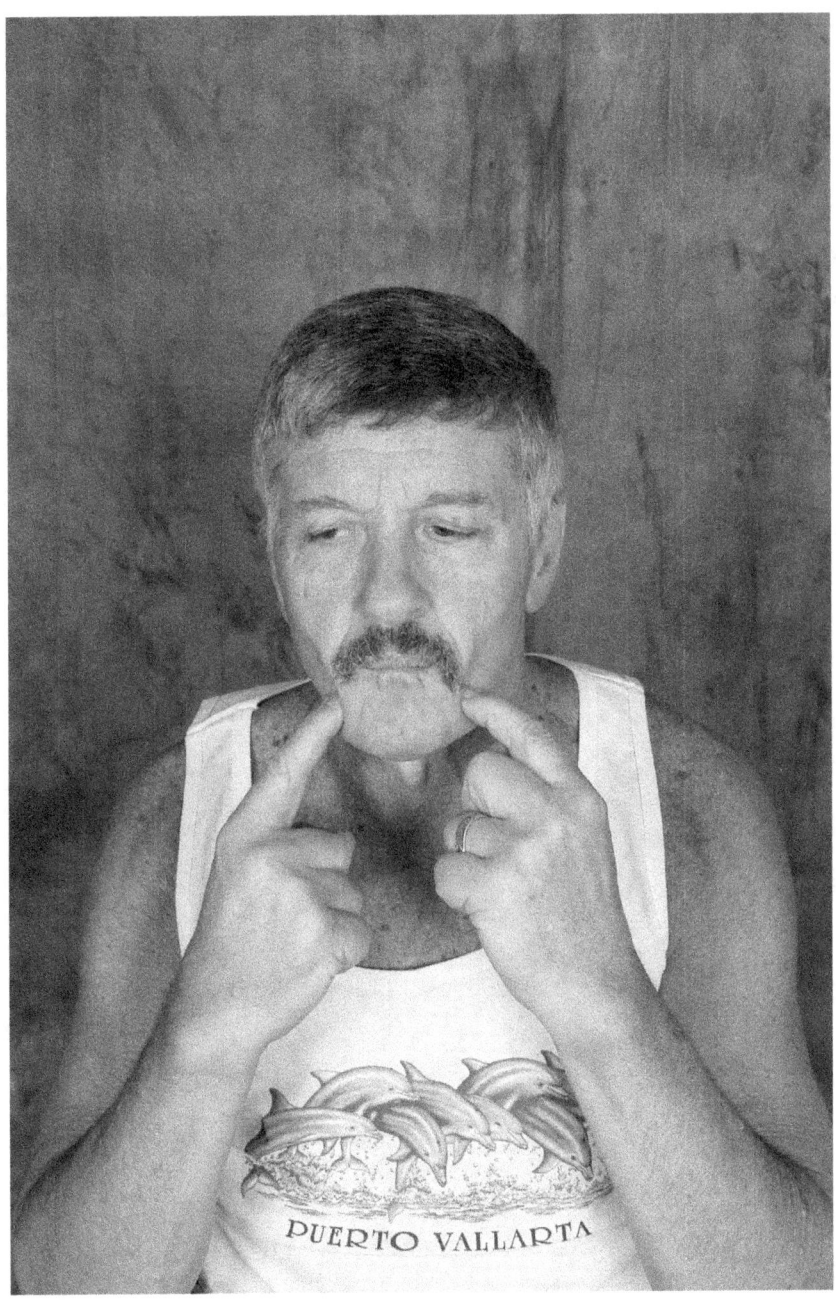

Figure 28

Two exercises you can do to stimulate the muscles in the face are to make the sound "OOOOOOOOOOO' and "EE-EEEEEE'.

I believe face massage is the most beneficial of all massages. It can leave the receiver looking 10 years younger and feeling stress free. Although wrinkles are an inevitable part of aging, massage can ease away fine lines so that your skin looks smoother and firmer, and it can help to prevent new lines from appearing. I call this routine a natural face-lift. You need to understand that by stimulating the muscle of the face, replacing the fat tissue and fiber with muscle makes this all possible.

CHAPTER X:

Regeneration Or Self Repair

Many animals have the ability to regenerate new appendages, like crabs growing new legs. Many arthropods molt, growing a new exoskeleton. Why can't humans repair themselves? I'm not saying we can grow new legs and arms, but we can repair organs, skin, cartilage, bones, muscles and ligaments. I can prove this statement. I already showed you how to stimulate new muscle growth.

Progenitor cells are the key. They are also called adult stem cells. These cells set up shop in the bone marrow. These adult stem cells retain the ability to grow into other kinds of cells. Why is this so exciting? Your own stem cells can be used to regenerate new tissue (like new skin when you sun burn your skin) to replace broken-down or diseased tissue and fix your own organs. Then you have the opportunity to reverse that aging process. I have three examples to prove that your body can repair itself.

Example one: I play a lot of golf. Hitting balls at the driving range for many hours a day. I developed a sore rotator cup which became very painful. At night when I lie on by right shoulder it was very noticeable. I had to sleep on my left side. I felt the rotator cup with my fingers and one part was very sore probably a tear. I applied pressure with my fingers to the sore area until the pain went away. I did this several times a day and the pain gradually went away. This process took about a year, (repaired rotator cup).

Example two: I had a sore knee; an old football injury. The inside of my right knee had a slight torn ligament. The problem became worse as I aged. The knee would make a clicking sound, had pain and the ligament would lock up. When I put pressure on the sore area with my index finger the pain would go away and the knee wouldn't make the clicking sound for a short period of time. So I decided to apply pressure to the sore area until the pain completely went away. I applied (strong) pressure for two or three minutes. The pain went completely away for the whole day. I thought the problem was completely solved, no more pain. That morning I couldn't get out of bed, my knee was so sore: I had to use my crutches for one day. After a week the pain went away, but I still had the same problems with the knee. So a couple of weeks later I decide to try this again, pressure, no pain, crutches, and pain for a week. But this time the knee completely repaired itself. Why did this happen? I think I stimulated the injured area by applying pressure. This sends a message to the stem cell to repair the injured area. All your cells have the ability to repair themselves throughout life. The problem is they must be stimulated to repair themselves. I have not read any material about self repair to injured areas. Is this a new discovery? I don't know. All I know is that my rotator cup and knee repaired themselves after pressure was applied.

Example three: My feet were very weak and had a lot of pain. By flexing and massaging my foot the pain went completely away. I run daily with no foot pain. If I have a sore area, I apply pressure to the area and the pain goes away.

At sixty I felt very weak and frail. Today at sixty six I feel very young and healthy. I no longer worry about dying. My goal is to live longer than any human has every lived and be healthy throughout this process. I could have waited until I was one hundred years old and still healthy and then write this book. But if I'm right!!! I would like other people to share this trip of a longer and healthy life.

Why should you read this book if you are young? Well, if you start this practice at an early age you could remain young forever and age at a much slower rate. Your body would not start losing its muscle mass at the age of 28 for males and 32 for females.

CHAPTER XI:
Reverse Arterial And Cardiovascular Aging

We have started to reverse the aging process of our muscle mass, by getting it closer to the original 50% mark through massaging and flexing. Simply stated, keeping your arteries and heart healthy and young is the second best thing you can do for your health. Keeping your arteries young helps you guard against heart attack, stroke, vascular disease, erectile dysfunction and helps prevent wrinkles.

It's this simple; nothing ages you faster than mistreating your heart and arteries. Conversely, nothing keeps you younger than taking care of your cardiovascular system, which is 90,000 miles in length.

Clogged arteries lack the ability to deliver blood to certain key areas, like the heart, brain, penis, and clitoris. This can cause problems which lead to heart attack, stroke, impotence, and decline of orgasm quality. Accelerated arterial aging can do damage to the peripheral nerves, and the development of vision problems that can cause blindness. We can fix all these problems.

Most of the premature aging your arterial system undergoes is a result of your lifestyle. You age yourself by not taking proper care of your body. Scientific data indicates that you can overcome years of bad choices and aging and make your arteries significantly younger. No matter what kind of life you've already led. Aging is reversible. You can have a "second chance" if you want it. If you perform a good habit for three years, the effect on your body is as if you've done it your entire life.

First, you must get a blood test. Then you must look at your blood test and see what problems you might have and how to fix these problems. Since these lab tests and the markers they reveal will be new to most of you, I feel it's important to tell you a little about them so that you can make sense of the result you get back. My hope is that by encouraging you to take the tests and by clarifying what it all means, it will help empower you to take charge of your heart and artery health, before it is too late.

The standard cholesterol test you get when you have a physical measures total cholesterol, LDL (bad cholesterol), HDL (good cholesterol), and triglycerides. Although you've almost undoubtedly had these tests done, you may not be sure what they really measure and how your test result correlates to your health.

I will talk you through the basic of each, explaining how each of these factors impacts your heart and circulatory system. The cutoff in the headings that follow, are the levels at which your numbers become unhealthy.

TOTAL CHOLESTEROL
Unhealthy result; 200 milligram or above

The standard measures the level of cholesterol in your blood. This is called your total cholesterol.

Cholesterol is needed in your body to produce cell membranes, hormones, and bile acids, as well as the material that helps keep skin moisturized. Cholesterol comes from two sources, our liver and the food we eat. You should keep your total cholesterol well below the cutoff, around 140 mg.

LDL CHOLESTEROL
Unhealthy result 130(mg), or above

LDL cholesterol the (bad) cholesterol carries cholesterol from the liver to cells in the body. High levels of it contribute to the risk of artery disease, and it is one of the primary markers used to predict coronary artery disease.

As LDL passes through the arteries, it can get trapped in already existing lesions. There, it's prone to oxidization, which further damages the arteries.

You can lower cholesterol by decreasing the amount of saturated fat you consume in food. Examples of foods high in saturated fats are meat, full-fat dairy products, lard, and coconut and palm oils. These are bad. In the nutrition chapter, I'll give you a list of foods that contain cholesterol so you can avoid them.

An LDL reading over 130 mg is unhealthy and should be considered an alert. You should try to keep your LDL "bad" cholesterol below 100.

OXIDATION: CREATING TOXIC LDL
The human body simply cannot survive without oxygen. But this life-giving element can also have a corrosive effect on the cells in our body. Kitchen science provides the clearest example of oxygen. When you cut an apple and leave it out, the exposure to the oxygen makes the flesh of the fruit turn brown. Chefs know that if you sprinkle the inside of the apple

with some lemon juice, the fruit will stay white. The vitamin C in the lemon juice acts as an antioxidant. It protects the apple's cells from the oxygen in the air.

How does this work on the arterial level? LDL, the "bad" cholesterol, becomes even more dangerous once it is oxidized. When LDL is oxidized, it becomes really desirable bait for the white blood cells that are working to repair the damaged artery wall. In an attempt to protect the body, the white blood cells eat more and more of these oxidized LDL particles in the arterial walls, until they become obese. The white blood cells turn into what's called a foam cell. This is because the fats inside of these cells have the appearance of foam. Foam cells die, are unstable, and prone to pop. When they pop, they coat the artery wall with foam. The foam hardens and calcifies the walls of the arteries. The walls become like a lead pipe. This is called arteriosclerosis. This disorder results in the narrowing and hardening of the arteries over time. Early in the arteriosclerosis process (hardening of the arteries), the diameter of the artery is not narrowed. The artery wall expands to accept the foam deposits, in the early stages of the disease. The blood flow is totally normal. Later, in the disease process, the artery can no longer expand. The only place left for the foam deposits to go is inward, blocking the flow of blood. Then, arterial plague builds up in calcified arteries. They are lethal. When the plaque ruptures, it can completely obstruct a partially blocked artery, causing a heart attack, stroke and even sudden death. Oxidation increases the likelihood of arterial damage, unstable plaque, and a cardiac event.

Obviously, we are looking to do anything we can to shore up the body's natural defenses against this process. The antioxidants in this plan are one way to do that. With the correct diet, the right supplements, and exercise, you can correct this problem.

Antioxidants help keep you from "rusting" on the cellular level. Certain foods and supplements are rich in antioxidants, and you can help protect yourself against the rusting process simply by eating the right foods and taking the right supplements. I'll give you a list foods and supplements in the nutrition chapter of this book.

HDL CHOLESTEROL.
Unhealthy result: 40 mg or below

HDL is called the (good) cholesterol because high levels of it are correlated to a reduced risk of artery disease. HDL removes cholesterol away from the artery walls, from plaque and carries it back to the liver for reprocessing, where it is either recycled or excreted. HDL also carries an important natural antioxidant enzyme. One that prevents the damaging oxidization of LDL cholesterol. You can raise HDL Cholesterol a number of ways: loss of excess body fat, vigorous exercise, and diet. I'll give you a list of foods which will increase your HDL. You should try to keep HDL above 50.

TRIGLYCERIDES
Unhealthy result: 140 (mg) or above

When you eat, your body converts extra energy into a form of energy that can be stored for later use. So calories get turned into fats, and when three of these molecules are bonded together, they're called triglycerides.

Triglycerides have been linked to artery disease, independent of LDL levels. High levels of triglycerides are strong predictors of heart attack. High triglycerides are problems when they're found in combination with high LDL cholesterol.

A good triglycerides reading would be around 65. Since diet is extremely important in controlling triglycerides, it's within most people's reach if they're paying attention to their diet. Since triglycerides can be the result of extra glucose in the blood, eating too many carbohydrates, simple sugars, alcohol and saturated fats can result in elevated levels. Losing excess weight can be powerful in controlling them. I'll give you a list of food which lowers your triglycerides in the nutrition chapter of this book.

HOMOCYSTEINE
Unhealthy result: 14 or above

Homocysteine is a naturally occurring substance. It is the by-product of the amino acid methionine. It's usually made after a meal rich in animal proteins. Methionine is mostly found in animal proteins, like chicken, pork, and beef. It's best to avoid those foods to lower homocysteine levels. Homocysteine levels seem to correlate to a higher risk of heart disease. One study by M.D. Rene Malinow showed that homocysteine levels lead to a three-time increase in the likelihood of having a stroke. Homocysteine is an abrasive that irritates the inside of the arteries. It makes it easier for LDL to move into the arterial walls. This process is called inflammation.

Inflammation of the arteries causes swelling of the artery walls. This constricts the arteries and reduces blood flow. Artery wall swelling also causes the blood flow to become turbulent. Turbulent blood flow causes potholes to form in the walls of the arteries. These potholes provide places where LDL (bad cholesterol) and white blood cells can seep into the wall of the artery creating plaque. The buildup of plaque reduces the diameter of the blood vessel and blood flow even more. A clot of plaque in a pothole can break off. It can travel to a smaller vessel in the heart, or brain, where it can cause major damage, like a heart attack or stroke by blocking the blood flow. The therapy for elevated homocysteine is to take B vitamins, including B6, B12 and folic acid. You must talk to your doctor before taking any kind of supplements.

CHAPTER XII:

The Diet Nutrition

Diet should be the first thing we seriously address when we want to get better. Unfortunately, it's no wonder that with all the effective medications that we have, doctors and patients are opting for pills over dietary changes to treat the symptoms of coronary and artery diseases. But, we should remember that diet itself is one of the most powerful tools in our battle against these diseases. Most cancers arise from or are promoted by our lifestyle choices, such as what we eat or don't eat. In fact, today we can do some amazing thing with diet.

The foods we eat are made up of building blocks-fats, carbohydrates, and protein. Those building blocks have fairly predictable effects on our bodies.

Grocery shopping is a crucial event. You need to know what you're going to be eating over the course of the week so you can shop in advance. Good food shopping helps you make sure your pantry and refrigerator stocked with healthy ingredients. Healthy, well stocked cabinets keeps you from ordering pizza deliveries, using drive-through heart attacks fast food establishments and buying spur of the moment foods that can age you.

FATS

Fats have long been cast as the number one artery-clogging, obesity-causing villains of American health. As a result, our supermarket shelves are bursting with low-fat and fat-free products.

The truth about fats, your body needs fat. Fat is the material in the cells that stores and provides energy; it protects us from the cold, and helps keep skin healthy. So our diets must have some fat in them.

What is a blood fat, the kind that's measured by the common blood test? It's a triglyceride. These fatty acids can be saturated and unsaturated fats. The difference between these fats on our arteries is dramatic. Fat isn't the enemy but the wrong kind of fat can be.

SATURATED FATS

Saturated fats are the "bad" fats. They'll raise your LDL "bad" cholesterol level more than anything else. No food element has been more closely linked to arterial aging than saturated fats. Saturated fats turn on certain genes that produce proteins associated with inflammation of blood vessels. This event is the first stage in developing cancer cells. Foods high in saturated fats promote plaque buildup along the artery wall, which is the first stage of cardiovascular disease and arterial aging.

Sources of saturated fat are beef, pork, lamb, chicken, whole-milk cheese, ice cream, whole milk, butter, cocoa butter, palm, and coconut oils.

Correct choices. Trim all visible fat off your meat. Choose lean cuts. When eating poultry choose white meat more often than dark meat and don't eat the skin. Choose low-fat or fat-free versions of your favorite dairy foods; nonfat or low-fat milk and cheese, ice milk or frozen yogurt instead of ice cream. Choose a canola-based tub margarine instead of butter. Avoid products containing tropical oil.

TRANS FATS

Food companies love to use trans fats in products because they give food a much longer shelf life. But trans fats
are not so good for your arteries. Trans fats not only raise
your LDL "bad' cholesterol. They also lower your HDL
"good' cholesterol. Major sources of trans fats are vegetable shortenings, margarines, hydrogenated peanut butter,
and commercially prepared baked goods such as pies, cakes,
cookies, crackers, pastries, doughnuts, potato chips and fast
foods.

Some experts estimate that as many as one-half of all cancers may be provoked, or their growth promoted, by our
dietary choices. Apparently, saturated and trans fats promote
the growth of cancer cells and the progression of cancer tumors. Other studies have noted a connection between fat
intake and a higher incidence of other types of cancers including lung cancer, lymphomas, ovarian, and prostate cancers.
Studies show that the more trans fat a person consumes, the
faster the cardiovascular system ages. Some researchers have
attributed as many as 50,000 deaths a year to trans fat consumption.

UNSATURATED FATS

Unsaturated fats are considerably better for you than saturated fats. There are actually two different types of unsaturated fats; monounsaturated and polyunsaturated. You should
make 25 percent of your calories or 20 grams healthy fat. You
need healthy fat for normal nerve and immune cell function,
and to make food taste great.

Monounsaturated fats, in contrast to saturated fats, help reduce the amount of bad cholesterol in the blood and boost the amount of good cholesterol, causing LDL levels to sink and HDL levels to rise. Major sources of monounsaturated fats are olive and canola oils. These fats are healthy-choice fats that you should be using at home for cooking and adding to foods. You can also find monounsaturated fats in walnuts and almonds. These nuts should not be roasted in oils or coated with flavorings. You may have read or heard about the Mediterranean diet, which relies heavily on olive oil, nuts, and other 'fatty' foods. These fats are mostly monounsaturated, which appears to account for the much lower coronary heart disease rates in countries that follow these diets.

The other kind of unsaturated fat is polyunsaturated fats. There are actually two important kinds of polyunsaturated fats; the omega-6s and the omega-3s.

The omega-6s fatty acids are found in vegetable oils such as corn, soybean, and safflower oils. The food industry uses a lot of these oils so you're probably already getting a lot of omega-6s in your diet. I suggest that you go lightly in your consumption of them. To do this is to make sure that they're not among the fats you use at home for cooking.

These omega-3s are nutrients that the body can't make on its own, so we need to get them from food. The best food source for these particular omega-3s is fish oil. Major sources are fish. Vegetable sources include canola oil, walnuts, flaxseed oils, wheat germ, and soybeans. Although the fatty acids found in the vegetable sources may not share the same benefits as the omega-3s found in fish. I recommend that you make fish a regular feature of your diet. Try for three fish meals a week, but add more if you'd like. Avoid deep-fried fish. Deep-fried fish is low in omega-3s and the fats these fish are fried in are generally high in unhealthy trans fats.

The omega-3s in fish and fish oils have been linked to reduced rates of coronary heart disease. They reduce triglycerides, raise HDL, and have other heart friendly side effects. They reduce the risk of blood clots and relax the arteries. They help regulate the electrical signals the heart muscle sends, decreasing the likelihood of irregular heart beat.

CARBOHYDRATES

Carbohydrates are the body's rapid source of energy. All carbohydrates are composed of sugar units. Chemically, carbohydrates can be classified as either simple or complex. Simple carbohydrates are commonly referred to as sugar. Think of this as fruit juices, dried fruit, soda, muffins, pies, cookies, etc. Complex carbohydrates are the starches and most fibers. Examples include whole grain products and pasta.

We can digest simple carbs more quickly than complex carbs. Sugars get absorbed into our bloodstream very rapidly and can cause a surge in blood sugar. This leads to a hormonal overcorrection, which dumps a ton of insulin into your bloodstream and may bring your blood sugar too low. That's why you feel an energy boost immediately after a sweet treat and feel ready for a nap about an hour later. Complex carbohydrates are absorbed into the bloodstream more slowly. In order to have the slowest, most even release of energy into your bloodstream, choose complex carbohydrates. Eat less from the simple carbohydrate category and more from the complex carbohydrate category. Make an effort to choose complex carbohydrate foods, such as legumes, barley, and most fruits and vegetables. Remember to have at least five servings of vegetables a day. Choose whole grains over white grains; multigrain bread over white; brown rice over white. Choose whole grain, unsweetened cereal over sugar cereal. Avoid excess sugar and products containing sugar. Sugar can increase our blood triglyceride levels. Complex carbohydrates generally don't increase triglyceride levels as much.

When you eat, your body converts extra sugars into a form of energy that can be stored for later use. So sugars get turned into fats, and when three of these fats are stuck together, they're called triglycerides. Triglycerides have been linked to both coronary and peripheral artery disease and higher levels of LDL (bad cholesterol). Since triglycerides can be the result of extra sugar in the blood, eating too many carbohydrates and simple sugars and drinking alcohol can result in elevated levels. Starchy vegetable, such as potatoes, are also high in simple carbohydrates. Avoid French fries at all cost.

The excess sugar we consume today develops into a syrupy mixture that coats our organs and creates glasslike shards that can cut up the blood vessels and tissues of our body. The constant wounds of these sugar surges lead to chronic inflammation. As a result, we're prone to infections and arterial damage and less able to cope with common stress we could normally fend off-like hypertension or high cholesterol, or even cigarette smoke.

PROTEIN

What is a protein? It's a chain of amino acids. The body contains 20 different kinds of amino acids. Proteins are the building blocks of the body's structures, such as your skin, organs, tendons, and muscles. Within each cell, proteins are constantly being made, without them; your body can't grow or heal.

Meat, eggs, and dairy products are very good sources of protein, but they can also be very bad sources of unhealthy saturated fats, which will increase your blood cholesterol, so don't forget to incorporate information about fat into your protein choices. Choose proteins that are low in saturated fat; fish, white meat skinless poultry, lean cuts of meat (once a week), egg whites, low fat dairy products, and low fat soy products. Whenever possible, replace meat with soy and high protein vegetable, like legumes.

CHOLESTEROL

Cholesterol isn't technically a building block, but since it's so central to all coronary heart disease, I'm going to talk about it in this section. Cholesterol does a lot of good things. Cholesterol is a basic building block for important hormones such as estrogen and testosterone, and it's an important component of cell structure. The problem starts when you have an abundance of LDL cholesterol which can promote arterial blockage.

Dietary cholesterol is found exclusively in animal products; eggs, meat and dairy products. Eggs and meats are the most concentrated sources of cholesterol.

For a long time, we warned people away from shellfish like oyster, clams, lobster, scallops, and crab because they were high in cholesterol. Now we know that they're actually all lower in cholesterol and contain very little fat. Shrimp, prawns, and squid are still high in cholesterol.

Wholesome choices. Choose egg-white products. Choose oysters, clams, crab, or lobster over shrimp and squid. Choose fat-free or low-fat versions of dairy products.

FIBER

Fiber is a key reason that diets high in fruit, vegetables, and grains are good for you. People who eat a lot of fiber have significantly lower rates of coronary heart disease. In countries where the diet is lower in fat and higher in fiber rates of coronary heart disease are lower. One of the explanations for this is that soluble fiber may block the reabsorption of cholesterol in the intestines. A person should eat at least 25 grams of fiber a day.

When you eat a steak, for example, molecules of fat and cholesterol pass through your intestinal wall and into your bloodstream and eventually get deposited as fat in your body. But before this can happen, fiber prevents you from absorbing these fats and calories. Fiber dissolves in your digestive tract, forming a sticky gel that acts like a protective coating, preventing fat and cholesterol from getting through your intestinal wall. Because fiber itself isn't absorbed, it passes out of your body, taking the fat and cholesterol with it! (keep a container of cleaned celery soaking in water in your refrigerator. After each meal eat a piece of celery. This will lower your cholesterol). The celery works like a statin drug. It will reduce your LDL, halt the buildup of plaque, and slash the danger of heart attack, stroke, erectile dysfunction, cancer, and death.

Fiber brings you many other benefits. They keep you regular. They lower your cholesterol and cut your risk of heart disease and neurological disorder in half. They can also reduce your risk of colon cancer by 30% because they sweep food particles out of your colon faster and keeps your insides cleaner.

Fiber is found solely in plant foods and is largely indigestible, passing through the digestive tract intact. Therefore, it contains no calories but makes you feel full sooner and helps control overeating.

It' not difficult to make a big difference through some minor modifications in your diet. All you have to do is to increase the number of whole grains, legumes, fruits, and vegetables in your diet. Choose whole wheat breads and pasta instead of their refined white alternatives. Make sure to eat at least five servings of vegetable a day. Add legumes to your soups and salads and a high-fiber cereal to your morning routine.

ALCOHOL

If you or your family members are not prone to alcohol abuse, one half to one drink of alcohol (beer, spirits, or wine) a day for women, and one to two drinks a day for men may be allowed. Some researchers believe that consuming alcohol in this manner is linked to higher overall "good" HDL cholesterol, reduction in death from coronary artery disease and have the lowest mortality rates.

A huge British study, reported in the Journal of the National Cancer Institute, found that as little as one alcoholic drink a day increases a woman's risk of several cancers, including breast cancer. That seemed to trump findings, going back decades, that moderate drinking can be a benefit by decreasing risk of heart disease.

The British study, far larger than ones done before, confirms earlier studies showing a link between drinking and breast cancer. The British researchers asked 1.3 million middle-age women about their drinking habits and followed their health for seven years. A single drink a day, they found, increased the risk for breast, liver and rectal cancer.

Medical research isn't simple; nor are medical decisions. Women at high risk for heart disease or cancer have better information than they did before to decide whether they'll have that glass of wine with dinner. They just need to decide which disease poses a bigger threat in their particular case.

CHAPTER XIII:

The Immune System

If you ask people what they fear the most when it comes to their health, many will say cancer, the second leading killer in the United States. In fact, cancer may soon pass heart disease and become number one. Cancer can be seen as a fact that your immune system is getting older and not protecting you from disease the way it should. Working to keep your immune system strong and young is the best way to safeguard yourself against a group of diseases. There are many lifestyle choices that will help keep you healthy, young, and cancer free.

Two types of cancer are prostate and breast cancer. Every year in the United States, about 250,000 new cases of prostate cancer are diagnosed, and 40,000 men die from this cancer. An estimated 210,000 new cases of breast cancer occur annually, and 40,000 women die from it. We have new tools to fight against cancer. What is important is that you realize that the ability of your immune system to do its job is directly related to how well you care for it. Despite the recent stir about cancer genes, fewer than 10 percent of all cancers are linked to genetic. We know that cancer is linked to lifestyle rather than heredity. Most cancers are promoted by our lifestyle choices, such as what we eat. Of course, smoking cigarettes is a well known culprit. Almost one-third of all cancers diagnosed is linked to tobacco use. But less commonly known is that food choices are thought to contribute to another third of cancers. People who eat diets low in saturated and trans fats, and rich in nutrients and healthy fat, have a significantly lower incidence of cancer. The choices in the food we eat, the amount of time we exercise, the hygiene we practice, the stress we undergo, and the otherwise imbalanced lives we lead account for about 65 percent of cancer deaths in the United States.

Clearly, we owe it to ourselves to avoid these cancers. What can we do to help avoid these diseases? The answer is as near as your kitchen. The good news is that the threat of these cancers that we fear can be reduced greatly with tomato (or spaghetti) sauce. Studies have shown that the risk of getting prostate cancer is as much as one-third lower among men who eat foods containing tomatoes or tomato paste as among men who rarely eat such foods. Similarly, studies have shown the risk of developing breast cancer is 30 to 50 percent lower among women who frequently eat foods containing tomatoes or tomato paste. These findings were backed by a study investigating a wide range of men in Hong Kong, Tokyo, Milan, New York and Chicago. The areas of the world having the lowest levels of prostate cancer are Mediterranean where tomato-based foods are central to the diet. Eat twelve tablespoon of low salt tomato sauce a week. Eat more ketchup and salsa. The carotenoid found in tomatoes, lycopene provides an immune strengthening antioxidant, anti-inflammatory falconoid that seems to inhibit growth of cancer, both prostate and breast, and make your arteries younger.

Carotenoids are also found in many fruits and vegetables. They have antioxidant and anti-inflammatory effects. You can spot them by the red, orange, green, and yellow colors found in many fruits and vegetables.

Flavonoids also provide antioxidants and inflammatory agents. They are found in plants. Flavonoids help you fight arterial and immune aging, and are plentiful in cranberries, cranberry juice, tea, tomatoes, apples, strawberries, blueberries, cherry, broccoli, onions, red wine, celery, grapes, and are found in colorful fruits and vegetables.

There are other strategies for the prevention of cancer, because it is far easier to prevent cancer than it is to cure it. Use good lifestyle choices to prevent cancer.

Sunlight helps our bodies produce an adequate amount of vitamin D. Vitamin D appears to strengthen the immune response and helps prevent certain kinds of cancers. Just ten to twenty minutes of sunlight a day is a healthy choice. Apply sun screen after absorbing ten to twenty minutes of sun rays. Unfortunately, many Americans live in areas where the sun isn't strong enough for them to get this benefit. A lot of these areas (North of North Carolina) won't get this benefit of the sun from October 1 to April 15. If you cannot get some sun every day, you should take 800 IU of vitamin D daily.

The truth is that simply flossing your teeth every day can actually make your arteries younger. The reason is that flossing helps keep your immune system young by preventing gum and periodontal infections. Bacteria that cause periodontal disease also trigger an immune response that causes inflammation of the arteries. Inflammation is the first stage of cancer. Studies show that the presence of periodontal disease, a disease most common in people with tooth loss, actually affects longevity. People who have gingivitis and periodontitis have a mortality rate 23 to 46 percent higher than those who don't floss their teeth daily.

The best behavior is to avoid cancer altogether. That means avoiding cancer-causing substances, such as avoiding nutrient deficiencies that lead to defects in repair process, and avoiding nutrients that increase the development of cancer cells. Eat nutrients that strengthen the immune system so that it can effectively destroy early cancer. Food choices, vitamins, exercise and prevention of stress are all keys to slowing aging of the immune system and keep us cancer free.

CHAPTER XIV:
Prostate Cancer

On March 30, 2006 I received my annual lab test results, following my yearly physical, and boy was I surprised!!! My prostate test (PSA) was 5.3, above 3.1 and you are looking at a possibility of cancer. I had a 25% chance of having prostate cancer. I had just turned 62 years old. I knew I was looking MR CANCER in the eye. This was really scary. I made an appointment to see my urologist. He ran a bunch of tests and did a biopsy to see if I had cancer. The results were negative. It wasn't at the cancer stage yet. I had to develop a plan of action. I wasn't going to get cancer if I had anything to do about it.

What was my plan of action? My Doctor didn't have a plan. He just told me to get an exam in six months and check my prostate again. I started to read a number of books on diet and the relationship of different foods to cancer. This is all the same information that I just explained to you. So, I changed my diet. I will give you examples of the types of foods I was eating and how these foods may have had something to do with my problem. I drank three or four cans of Coke a day. I loved pink and white candy coated licorice, (three bags a week). I loved ice cream (a gallon a week), three or four cookies a day, pork and beef five times a week. Fast food hamburgers and French fries with a large shake were part of my diet twice a week. You get the point? I had a very bad diet. My blood test revealed this: cholesterol 238, triglycerides 180, HDL 34, LDL 190, PSA 5.3, all these results where abnormal.

I decided to start eating a healthy diet. This is an example of the types of food I started eating. Breakfast; eat whole wheat cereal, banana, grapes, and almonds. Lunch; sandwich, which contain two slices of wheat bread, light canola cholesterol free mayonnaise, mustard with turmeric, tomato ketchup, sliced tomato, thin sliced chicken breast and a piece of fruit. Dinner; salad, cooked vegetables, chicken breast or some type of fish four to six times a week. I would make a large pot of spaghetti using wheat pasta and loaded with vegetables. This can be used during the week when you don't have time to cook a meal. Snacks; vegetables should be cut and ready to grab in a container on the top shelf in the refrigerator. Put fruit in a bowl on the counter so you see it right away. Get rid of the junk foods that tempt you!

Shopping is a crucial step, and you need to know what you're going to be eating over the course of the week so you can shop in advance.

On 3/27/07 I received my annual physical results. The lab results where amazing. Cholesterol 156, Triglycerides 40, HDL 99, LDL 99, Prostate test (PSA) .8. My plan really worked!! No more cancer to worry about! I changed my diet and rid myself of prostate cancer.

I have read other articles with the same results. Jim was diagnosed with prostate cancer. They told him that with no medical intervention, he had one year to live. They predicted that if he had his prostate removed and went through a chemotherapy and radiation treatment regimen, he might last 4 to 5 years. Instead of undergoing these changes, he changed his lifestyle. He started researching and learned that saturated and trans fat increased the growth of prostate cancer, and that lycopene and selenium decrease growth of these cells. He learned all about nutrition. He learned which foods contain fiber, about the value of whole grains over processed food, about fruits and vegetables, and about healthful fats. He changed his diet and as a consequence has done away with his cancer. I believe that all or most cancers are related to your diet and that by controlling your diet it will reduce the chance of you getting cancer. This will strengthen the immune system so that it can effectively scavenge early cancers.

THE ANTICANCER LIFESTYLE

A physician and neuroscience researcher discovered that he had a cancerous brain tumor at the age of 31. Being a physician didn't protect him from cancer, but it allowed him to dig deeply into the medical literature in search of ways to live longer than the few years he was expected to survive.

The first thing he learned is that we all carry cancer cells in us, even if only a few. But we also have natural defenses that usually prevent these cells from becoming an aggressive disease. These defenses include our immune system; the bodily functions that control inflammation; and foods that reduce the growth of blood vessels needed by tumors.

More than one third of Americans will develop detectable cancer. But nearly two thirds will not; their natural defenses will have kept the disease from taking hold. To survive his brain cancer, he knew, he needed to learn how to strengthen his own protective systems. We don't get cancer by genetics alone. A study in The New England Journal of Medicine found that people who were adopted at birth had the cancer risk of their adoptive parents rather than that of their biological parents. At most, genetic factors contribute 15 percent to our cancer risk. What determines the other 85 percent of our risk is what we do-or do not do enough of-with our lives.

When it comes to surviving cancer once it is diagnosed, there are no proven substitutes for conventional treatments: Surgery, chemotherapy, radiotherapy, or immunotherapy. These treatments target the tumor: By killing the tumor cells. They do not help prevent the disease, and they do not help keep it from coming back.

For prevention it is important to change the environment that surrounds cancer cells. Research suggests that cancer grows much faster under three circumstances: When a person's immune system is weakened and less capable of destroying budding tumors. When low-grade chronic inflammation in the body supports the invasion of neighboring tissue. When tumors are allowed to develop new blood vessels to feed growth.

When we boost the immune system, reduce inflammation, and reduce the growth of new blood vessels, we help create an anticancer environment. Research demonstrates the lifesaving result. At Ohio State University, a team followed women with breast cancer who all had surgery and conventional treatment. Some participated in an education group focused on better nutrition, more exercise, and stress release. Those who learned to change their lifestyle were half as likely to die from their cancer during the 11-year study as those who did not. This research shows that lifestyle choices can transform the body's ability to resist cancer.

So what are these cancer-fighting behaviors? Stress causes inflammation and weakens your immune system. Though we can't avoid stress in our lives, we can learn to respond to it differently and reduce our level of stress hormones. Practices such as yoga and meditation can reduce stress and strengthen our resistance to disease.

Regular physical activity has been shown to improve survival rates for many types of cancer. Just walking briskly for 30 minutes, seven times a week, dramatically reduces the chances of getting cancer.

Sugar and other foods (already mentioned in the book) fuels inflammation and cancer growth. Avoid these foods. Adding known cancer fighter such as herbs and spices: Mint, thyme, sage, turmeric, basil, and ginger. Foods rich in omega-3 fatty acids: Salmon, walnuts, sardines, and mackerel. Vegetables like: Broccoli, cauliflower, cabbage and (others that were mentioned in the book). Add berries, dark chocolate, and beverages such as: Green tea, pomegranate juice, water and red wine in moderation.

Though they can't be avoided completely, common household toxins should be minimized. Substances that can impair your body's cancer-fighting system include certain preservatives in cosmetics (called parabens and phthalates). Teflon released from scratch pans and high heat when cooking. Gases given off by new polyvinyl chloride objects such as those used in plumbing pipes, and biphenyl A from water heated in hard plastics.

As a physician who has now been living with cancer for 16 years, he discovered that we can all make our bodies tougher targets for cancer through the choices we make in our lives. As strange as it may seem, he is in better health than before he became ill.

Most people who start on this health journey notice a difference within a few months. Recent studies suggest that a healthy habit can have an impact on cancer statistics within a year or two. Another example how your diet and lifestyle can affect your life.

CHAPTER XV:

Erectile Dysfunction

At the age of 49 my love life was great. I had no problem and enjoyed sex daily, but in one year all this was going to change. During these 49 years, my diet was very poor and I plugged up my arteries with cholesterol and plaque. I remember the exact date I developed erectile dysfunction, June the first. My lovely wife wanted to make love and I couldn't stand at attention. This problem went on for three weeks. So I made a call to my doctor and he gave me the magic pill. No more problems, everything worked great. But was this the right answer? My doctor didn't explain why I had this problem. He just gave me the pill. Could this problem be solved in a different way? At the age of sixty six I no longer have this problem, because I changed my diet. I did some research on this subject of ED and I will share these results with you. By the way, the diet is one way to correct this problem. I went on a healthy diet and my arteries started to reduce the plaque buildup. In one year the ED started to get better. Three years later I no longer have ED. I explained my diet in the prostate chapter.

The magic pills have many side effects and I would like to share some of the results I have experienced. The pill can cause headache, high blood pressure three to five days after taking the pill, increased pulse rate, blurred vision, and depression. Other effects are that it can cause indigestion, flushing of the face, nasal stuffiness, mild back pain, and muscle pain.

If you have an eye condition which affects your retina you should discuss taking the magic pill with your doctor before taking it. If you experience any sudden loss of vision while taking the pill then stop taking the pill and talk to your doctor.

Are these pills safe? No. And are these effects life threatening? The answer is yes. I experienced irregular heart beat. This lasted for three days. The heart would beat three times and skipped a beat. I didn't call a doctor because I knew what caused the problem. The beat became normal again after the pills effect wore off.

The doctor will give you the pill if you are one percent healthy. How safe is this? How many health problems have occurred by taking the pill? Is a heart attack or stroke really worth it?

Erectile dysfunction is the inability to get and keep an erection sufficient for satisfactory sexual activity. Studies found that 52% of men aged 40 to 70 years had some degree of ED. Age was an important factor in ED: Approximately 40% of men aged 40 years versus 70% of men aged 70 years reported mild, moderate or severe ED. Every year, more than 600,000 new cases of ED are diagnosed in the United States alone.

However, age alone does not explain the increased risk for ED. As you age, you are also at greater risk for medical conditions that can be associated with ED, such as high blood pressure, cardiovascular (heart) disease, high cholesterol, and diabetes. In fact, any condition that narrows or hardens the blood vessels can cause ED. This is because erections require good blood flow into the erection chambers in the penis or clitoris. If the arteries are blocked or diseased, blood flow will be reduced causing some degree of ED. Use of some drugs can also lead to Ed. If you have recently started taking a new medication and suddenly notice difficulty attaining erections, you should speak with your doctor about possibly switching to another drug.

Depression, anxiety, stress, or relationship difficulties can also be an important cause of ED. Similarly cigarette smoking, physical inactivity, and being overweight or obese can all contribute to ED. Luckily, these are all conditions or choices over which you have some degree of control.

Not all ED is caused by a medical condition. You might notice that when you are particularly stressed at work, or very tired, or are having a rough spell with your partner, you have more difficulty having an erection. If you notice that you have strong morning erections, but cannot keep an erection during intimacy, develop ED suddenly or have ED intermittently, your problem may be psychological. Your doctor might recommend that you make an appointment to talk with a psychologist, or sex therapist.

If fear of lung cancer is not a sufficient incentive to help you to quit smoking, here is a great motivator: Smoking cigarettes has been associated with ED. Cigarette smoking can cause plaque to build-up in your arteries-including your penile or clitoral arteries. Nicotine can impair arterial blood flow into the penis or clitoris. According to information from the American Heart Association, smoking 20 cigarettes per day increases your risk of ED by 60% compared to men and women who never smoked. Therefore, stopping cigarette smoking can help to prevent ED.

There may be a relationship between being overweight or obese and having ED. One study found the prevalence of overweight or obesity in men with ED may be as high as 79%. This study also found that reducing your total body weight by at least 10% over a 2 year period, through "diet"!!! And physical activity, can substantially improve your erectile function. Men who remain physically active have a lower risk of ED than men who are sedentary. Thus, increasing your level of physical activity will reduce your risk of ED. Results found that men who had been sedentary but who initiated physical activity during middle-age significantly reduced their risk of ED.

Alcohol initially acts as a stimulant, but quickly becomes a central nervous system depressant that can temporarily interfere with your erectile capacity. Long-term alcohol abuse can also interfere with your desire for sex, and can interfere with your body's ability to send messages through the nervous system from your brain to your penis or clitoris. Reducing your alcohol consumption is important for many reasons, including the potential benefits to your sexual life.

Erectile dysfunction need not be a necessary part of aging. There are many simple changes you can make today to help maintain your sexual functions throughout the rest of your life. The messages to keep your heart healthy are exercise each day, eat well, stop smoking, and don't overindulge-will also help keep your sex life healthy.

CHAPTER XVI:
Supplements

I believe we need supplemental vitamins, minerals, and antioxidants because our bodies do not produce all these nutrients, so they must come from an outside source. A supplement is anything taken to increase the amount of nutrients in the diet. The body doesn't make its own vitamins, antioxidants and minerals. It takes what it needs from the foods we eat. If the foods that we eat don't supply enough of these things or, if some aspect of our lives overtaxes our supply of those things, supplements can be taken to make up for the deficiency.

Antioxidants are considered among the most crucial elements of vitamins. To understand antioxidants, oxygen is necessary for our bodies to function at all. Once it enters your cells, oxygen forms the basis of many of the cells most fundamental processes. This same oxygen in the form of unstable ions called free radicals can oxidize tissues. Oxygen waste products build up in organs such as the heart and brain, leaving brown discoloration on the tissues. This may be a more fundamental problem such as inflammation that causes IMMUNE DYSFUNCTION. These brown spots are sign of aging. The older you get, the more prevalent they become. If you slice an apple and leave it out in the air, it will soon turn brown. Exposed to air, the surface of the apple oxidizes. This process is similar to what happens when oxygen radicals build up in your body. If you were to take that apple and sprinkle lemon juice on the slices, they would stay white, because lemon juice is full of vitamin C, which works as an antioxidant.

Free radicals are temporarily unstable atoms or molecules with extra or unpaired electrons, which react with other atoms or molecules to produce another unstable molecule. Free radicals can cause inflammation and can damage our organs and DNA; they cause premature aging of the cells and promote cancers. Our body can get rid of them when antioxidants and some other molecules bind with unstable free radicals to make them neutral or stable. Then, they can be washed harmlessly out of the body in urine.

I'd like to begin our discussion of supplements with a warning. There's a common misconception that vitamins, minerals, and herbs are harmless simply because they're "natural" products. This simply isn't true. While these supplements can be very effective in affecting your health, they can also be toxic in the incorrect dosage, they can react badly with other medications you're taking, and they can have harmful effects on other aspects of your health.

I recommend taking a baby aspirin every day if there are no medical problems. If you are at risk for coronary heart disease you should talk to your doctor to find out if he or she thinks it's a good idea for you. Aspirin works to decrease your blood's tendency to clot. Platelets are components in your blood that aid in clotting your blood. That's ordinarily a good thing; it prevents you from bleeding to death from a cut. Blood clots that get stuck around the plaque in the arteries, are a major cause of heart attack. So it benefits people to decrease platelets clotting. Aspirin reduces the blood's clotting tendency by poisoning some of those platelets.

Aspirin also acts as an anti-inflammatory. Since inflammation contributes to coronary heart disease by weakening the fatty buildup inside the arterial walls, causing rupture and blood clots, taking anti-inflammatory measures may be a good way to prevent heart attack and stroke.

The antioxidant defense plan, in this plan: the two supplements that we use are vitamin C and vitamin E. They can prevent oxidation which is one of the first steps in the formation of atherosclerosis (hardening of the arteries) and unstable plaque. The more vitamin E there is within the LDL particle, the more resistant it is to oxidative damage. That's a good thing, since oxidized LDL can be so lethal. The Cambridge Heart Attack and Antioxidant Study showed that men with coronary heart disease who took vitamin E showed a significant reduction in nonfatal heart attacks. This study strongly suggested that vitamin E is beneficial if you already have coronary heart disease.

You remember the example of the cut apple flesh that turns brown unless sprinkled with lemon juice. In that case, it's the vitamin C in the lemon juice that protects the apple flesh from oxidization. Vitamin C is one of our most powerful antioxidants. Take 400 IU of vitamin E once a day and 500 milligrams of vitamin C twice a day.

The use of fish oil for many years has also been shown to lower very high triglycerides. Fish oils have also been used to help treat high blood pressure. They may help to prevent irregular heartbeats. Fish oil helps to maintain the elasticity of the artery walls. They help stabilize plaque that might otherwise have the potential to rupture. Fish oil promotes heart health. Take 1,000 to 2,000 mg of fish oil a day. The Oslo Study Diet which was done in 1,200 men showed that fish oils promote heart health.

Homocysteine is a naturally occurring by- product of the amino acid methionine, which is made by the body in the process of digesting food, especially meat. Most people don't have a problem with this homocysteine. They eat some meat, their homocysteine levels rise, and their bodies automatically flush the residual levels out of their bloodstreams. Some people inherit either a compromised ability or a complete inability to clear it from their bloodstream, so their levels remain high. Homocysteine itself is irritating to the inside of the arteries, acting almost like a piece of sandpaper. This not only causes inflammation but irritates the surface, making it easier for the other factors that cause coronary heart disease to worm their way into the arterial wall to do their damage.

So if you have inherited this inability to adequately clear homocysteine from your blood then your body will need additional support to get the job done and this is where the B vitamins come in. The B vitamins are cofactors for the enzymes that foster this homocysteine-clearing process. So taking the appropriate B vitamins to supercharge those enzymes can help to compensate for an inherited inefficiency in clearing homocysteine naturally. Take 2 micrograms of foliate acid, 250 milligrams of B6, and 10,000 units of B12. These doses must be guided by your physician.

Vitamin D is unique among essential nutrients because we get very little of it from food. Instead, our bodies make it when the sun's ultraviolet rays activate a chemical in our skin that is used to synthesize the nutrient. It's long been known that D helps our bones absorb calcium, but that turns out to be far from its only critical function. The stunning discovery of vitamin D receptors in almost every tissue and organ suggests that our muscles, nerves, and even our immune systems need D for peak performance. Because we don't get enough sun, we have evolved into a species that does not meet its vitamin D needs naturally. It's not surprising that 25 different studies that looked at blood levels of vitamin D in a variety of populations revealed widespread insufficiency noted Michael Holick, MD, of Boston University. His research showing insufficient levels in 40 to 100 percent of elderly Americans and Europeans.

Vitamin D is safe in much higher doses than first thought, too. "There were no controlled safety studies 10 years ago when we set the recommendations, so upper limits were kept pretty low. Now, several good clinical trials show safety at 10,000 IU or more," says Robert Heaney, MD, the Creighton University researcher. According to recent findings, vitamin D can help do the following.

Increase your odds of living longer. Research published recently in Archives of Internal Medicine that combined 18 studies of 57,000 people, mostly middle-aged or elderly, showed those who took any supplemental dose of vitamin D from 300 to 2,000 IU (mostly 400 to 800 IU) were 7 percent less likely to die for any reason over the length of the studies than those who took no supplement. There were no negative side effects from the supplements.

Fend off falls and fractures. Several studies have shown that taking calcium and vitamin D helps the elderly have fewer of the falls and fractures that can lead to prolonged hospitalization and even death.

Increase cancer resistance. Starting around Atlanta, the farther north you go (where year-round sun is weaker), the greater your risk of developing non-Hodgkin's lymphoma and colon, pancreatic, breast, and prostate cancers. Studies also show that lower blood levels of vitamin D are associated with a 30 to 50 percent increased risk of both getting and dying of colon, prostate, or breast cancer. Though we don't yet know why, Dr. Welsh's new research shows that higher levels of vitamin D can prevent, slow, and kill breast cancer cells in lab dishes and animals.

Ease chronic pain. Young women often have nonspecific bone and muscle pain and supplementing with vitamin D brings great relief. 25 percent of the patients who have had chronic pain for years turn out to be vitamin D deficient. Vitamin D deficiency doesn't cause the pain but it does contribute to the discomfort. So taking supplements will ease the chronic pain, noted Michael Hooten ,MD, director of the Pain Rehabilitation Cent of the Mayo Clinic.

Other large studies suggest that vitamin D deficiency puts you at risk for arthritis, multiple sclerosis, type 2 diabetes, depression, and even dental problems. All experts agreed that a supplement of 800 to 1,000 IU is safe for everyone except those with a rare absorption disorder.

Calcium and magnesium is for strong bones and calm nerves. You probably know that you need calcium for strong teeth and bones, but you may not be aware that you need this essential mineral for the proper functioning of every one of your trillions of cells. Studies show that calcium can help preserve your bones into old age. This is a very good thing if you want to walk, not roll, through the door to your ripe old age.

Magnesium works with calcium to build proteins, produce energy, and support good nerve function. Supplementation can help with poor sleep, anxiety, menstrual and muscle cramps or spasms, high blood pressure, asthma attacks, and abnormal heartbeats. Take 400 mg magnesium and 700 mg of calcium twice a day.

Coenzyme Q 10: could it be the fountain of youth? Because CoQ-10 levels often decline in your body as you age, some researchers have proposed that CoQ-10 may be helpful in slowing the aging process.

CoQ-10 functions to help the cells of your body produce energy in the mitrochondria-the power center of the cell. It works specifically in the cells of your nervous system found in the heart, nerves, and brain.

CoQ-10 acts as an antioxidant protecting tissues (especially heart tissues) from free radical damage, radical oxygen molecules that attack your cells. It also acts as an immune supporter by regulating immune processes, an energy enhancer by enhancing the manufacture of energy molecules in your cells, and a cancer-fighting substance. Some published studies on this supplement show size reduction in breast cancer tumors.

Use this coenzyme (a substance needed for the function of enzymes) in conjunction with exercise and weight loss programs because it is one of nature's most potent antioxidants, cell-growth regulators, and energy-enhancing substances. It can also protect against diabetes and cardiovascular problems, including arrhythmia, cardiomyopathy (enlarged heart), congestive heart failure, and hypertension.

CoQ-10 is also potentially useful in treating many other symptoms and diseases, such as tinnitus (ringing in the ears), senility and Alzheimer's disease, male infertility and low sperm counts, and general fatigue.

According to reports, CoQ-10 can decrease your response to Coumadin, a blood-thinning drug. Consult your doctor before using CoQ-10 in conjunction with pharmaceutical drugs for serious ailments. The usual dose is 200 mgs a day 100 in the morning and 100 in the evening.

Flaxseed oil is probably the most balanced vitamin and nutritious oil. This is because it contains both omega-3 and omega-6 fatty acids. Flaxseed is cancer-protective because they help stabilize cell membranes and structures, and also offer cardio-protective benefits. Flaxseed is bowel toners to keep your system moving smoothly. Suggested amounts are two to four teaspoons, up to two tablespoons per day, or two to four capsules of flaxseed oil.

Glucosamine sulfate, or just glucosamine, is a raw material needed by your body to make substances that your joints use to build and maintain cartilage, as well as repair damaged cartilage. Glucosamine is perhaps the most popular dietary supplement for easing the symptoms of osteoarthritis. It may also prove helpful for speeding the healing of wounds and to reduce symptoms of some gastrointestinal disorders. Start with 500 mg of glucosamine sulfate three times daily; for acute joint pains, you can take 1,000 mg three times a day, without any side effects. You may find that higher dosages taken less frequently are more effective, but two or three weeks are necessary before you'll notice its benefits.

Chondroitin sulfate is one of the materials in substance that heal your joints, but no one has proved that it's readily absorbed from the human intestines, and we aren't certain that it's an active ingredient in these joint- healing formulas. You can take 400 mg of chondroitin sulfate three times a day.

Saw palmetto has become well known in recent years because of its effectiveness in reducing the symptoms of prostate inflammation and enlargement. It strengthens the urinary and genital organs, helping to relieve burning or incomplete urination and reduced urinary flow. Traditional uses also include strengthening the female or male reproductive tract and restoring sexual vitality. Take 1 capsule twice daily. But in addition take 1 or 2 extra capsules per day. A higher dose is more effective.

Garlic in recent years, due to positive clinical results, practitioners have begun recommending garlic for high blood pressure and high cholesterol. Clinical trials have also confirmed garlic's anti-fungal activity in treating Candida. You can purchase deodorized capsules and tablets of garlic from natural foods store. Follow direction on the label regarding dosage.

In general, if you eat a balanced and healthy diet, with four servings of fruits, five servings of vegetables, and plenty of grains, you should get all the nutrients you need through your food. However, most of us have busy lives and hectic schedules, which means that it's not always easy to eat a balanced and nutrient rich diet. I recommend taking a multivitamin every day in case you have missed out on a little bit of one mineral or the other.

What is fish oil? Omega-3-Fatty Acids are one of two groups of fatty acids which the body cannot make but which are essential for normal growth and development. Fish oil contains EPA (eicosapentaenoic acid) and DHA (docosahexaenoic acid). Both EPA and DHA are known as essential omega-3 fatty acids because the body cannot make them on its own.

Thousands of people die from heart attack each year. Might something as simple and readily available as fish oil prevent some of these deaths? Many doctors, nutritionists and researchers believe so.

Omega-3 oils (fish oils) protect the heart by preventing blood clots or keeping other fats from injuring the arterial walls. They not only relax arteries but also help to decrease constriction of arteries and thickening of blood. Data suggests that omega-3 fatty acids may reduce the risk of cardio-vascular-related death by 29–52%. The risk of sudden cardiac death among those who consumed higher levels of omega-3 via fish oil was found to be reduced by 45–81%. Fatty acid intake also significantly reduced plasma cholesterol and triglyceride levels. Fish oil is a naturally occurring substance and is considered by many experts to be a safe and effective treatment for patients who have had a heart attack.

There is now clear evidence that dietary supplementation of omega-3 fatty acid is essential for normal eye and brain development. This is especially crucial for infants.

Research on mice has shown that EPA supplementation inhibits tumor growth. EPA or omega-3 acids from fish oil have also been used to treat Crohn's disease, rheumatoid arthritis, and kidney disease. EPA has also been shown to help regulate and maintain a healthy immune response.

I have had tinnitus (ringing in the ears) for many years. At times, I noticed that this ringing sound would disappear. Within the last year (2008), I figured out how to stop this ringing sound and I no longer have this problem. I will share this information with you and maybe this will cure any tinnitus problem you might have. The information involves supplements and diet.

A common cause of tinnitus is inner ear cell damage. Tiny, delicate hairs in your inner ear move in relation to the pressure of sound waves. This triggers ear cells to release an electrical signal through a nerve from your ear (auditory nerve) to your brain. Your brain interprets these signals as sound. If the hairs inside your inner ear are bent or broken, they can "leak" random electrical impulses to your brain, causing tinnitus.

Eating right and taking other steps to keep your blood vessels healthy can help prevent tinnitus linked to blood vessel disorders.

Step 1: A diet high in simple carbohydrates produces a large amount of cholesterol and glucose which will junk up the tiny, delicate hairs in your inner ear causing tinnitus. I found that when I would eat a diet high in simple carbohydrates, I would experience ringing ears. Having a diet with complex carbohydrates and eating only chicken and fish will help prevent this problem.

Step 2: By taking 30 mg of CoQ-10 and 2,000 mg of fish oil, my problem was solved. I hope this works for you.

You should really take your multivitamin twice a day: Several vitamins are water soluble and you will urinate them out so quickly that you need them twice a day just to have a minimally acceptable level in your blood at all times (especially if you do not eat a lot of fruit and vegetables). Further, for some nutrients such as calcium, you cannot absorb more than 600 mg at a time: Vitamin C, you cannot absorb more than 500mg at a time. You want a twice-a-day multivitamin. Although many may be unwilling to take their vitamins twice a day, that is the optimal way for health.

CHAPTER XVII:

Alzheimer's

Dementia about one-third of the population over age 80 show symptoms of dementia, which may include a loss of memory for recent events, neglect of appearance, and repeated question while ignoring replies or answers. In later stages, victims may become both bedridden and incontinent. Symptoms of dementia may appear as early as age 60 in one type of Alzheimer's.

About 55 percent of dementia cases are the result of early or late onset Alzheimer's disease. But in both cases brain damage occurs due to the abnormal production of the protein plaque amyloid.

Brain tissue taken from a person afflicted with Alzheimer's disease reveals a deposit of a protein called amyloid plaque, which is a typical feature of the disease. Another main feature is a tangle of filaments within the brain's gray matter.

About 15 percent of the people who are affected by Alzheimer's have brain damage that is caused by a series of lacunar strokes. Many blood vessels become blocked over a period of several years, due to diet.

Amyloidosis is a group of diseases that result from the abnormal deposition of a particular protein, called amyloid, in various tissues of the body. Amyloid protein can be deposited in localized area of the body. Amyloidosis that affects tissues throughout the body is referred to as systemic amyloidosis. Systemic amyloidosis can cause serious changes in virtually any organ of the body. Amyloidosis can occur as a result of another illness, including chronic infections, or chronic inflammatory diseases. Amyloidosis can also be localized to a specific body area. The protein that deposits in the brain of patients with Alzheimer's disease is a form of amyloid.

Amyloid plaques are found in widespread areas of the brain, including in the cerebral cortex, hippocampus, basal ganglia, thalamus, and even the cerebellum. Thus, Alzheimer's disease appears to be a metabolic degenerative disease. Alzheimer's disease is an excess accumulation of amyloid plaque. A blood protein that transports cholesterol to the tissues, has accelerated deposition of amyloid and thus greatly increased the risk for Alzheimer's disease, due to diet. No cure has been found and some drugs may slow the progression for only very limited time periods.

Can you prevent Alzheimer's? Can you stop the spreading of the disease, neutralize it or even put it into prolonged remission? I don't have a cure for Alzheimer's, but I think I can prevent you from getting it, and if you have it you can put it into prolonged remission with the correct diet.

Vascular disorder may contribute to progression of Alzheimer's disease. There is also accumulating evidence that cerebrovascular disease caused by hypertension (high blood pressure) and arteriosclerosis (hardening of the arteries) may play a role in Alzheimer's disease. Cerebrovascular disease is the second most common cause of acquired cognitive impairment and dementia and likely contributes to cognitive decline in Alzheimer's disease. In fact, many of the common risk factors for cerebrovascular disease, such as hypertension, diabetes, and hyperlipidemia (high cholesterol), are also recognized, to greatly increase the risk for developing Alzheimer's disease.

Reducing high blood pressure to normal (120 over 80) improves cognitive function and slows Alzheimer's progression substantially. If you have high blood pressure, then you have a five times greater risk of getting dementia two decades down the line. If you have elevated blood pressure, it may be because your arteries are constricted, often as a result of cholesterol plaques, (high cholesterol), and limit the amount of blood and nutrients that reach a particular area. In the case of the brain, not having sufficient blood supplied (blocked arteries) is what elevates the risk of lacuna stroke. This can happen throughout the brain. A lack of healthy blood flow to the brain is one of the main causes of forgetfulness or dementia. All this can be controlled by diet.

Aging of your arteries is caused by both high blood pressure and high blood sugar. High blood sugar cause nicks or holes in the arteries walls of the brain that trigger the destructive process of inflammation and result in atherosclerosis. Atherosclerosis process is the deposit of fats in the inner walls of the arteries of the brain. These waxy deposits are called plaque (amyloid) and made up of a combination of fats, cholesterol, and scar like tissue. These plaque deposits reduce the diameter of the inside of the artery, thereby reducing blood flow. Clogged arteries lack the ability to deliver blood to certain key areas, like the brain. Atherosclerosis increases the inflammation that ages the brain cells. A little physical activity and diet can dramatically improve the ability of insulin to get glucose (sugar) into many cells, especially muscle, reducing the chances of getting atherosclerosis.

Glucose in the blood and normally you have a very tight junction between the endothelial cells (a single layer of smooth, thin cells which line the blood vessels) in your arterial wall is that, nothing can get between them. Glycosylation weakens that junction between cells and make them leak and vulnerable to tears. Excess glucose in the blood is like glass cutting artery and even organs. The body repairs those tears by plugging them with cholesterol, which causes plague and inflammation in your arterial walls of the brain.

If glucose can't get into a cell, it stays in the blood and gunks up the proteins in our brain. It damages the things it touches. Now the body must clean up this mess. This process is chemotaxis. When a tissue becomes inflamed, at least a dozen different products are formed that can cause chemotaxis toward the inflamed area in the brain. Chemotaxis depends on the concentration gradient of the infected area. The concentration is greatest near the source which directs the movement of the white blood cells. The most important function of the neutrophils and macrophages is phagocytes, which means cellular ingestion of the offending agent. Phagocytes must be selective of the material that is phagocxtized; otherwise normal cells and structure of the brain might be ingested.

Whether phagocytes will occur depends especially on two selective procedures. First, most natural structures in the tissues have smooth surfaces, which resist phagocytosis (ingestion of tissue). If the surface is rough, the likelihood of phagocytosis is increased in the brain.

Second, most natural substances of the body have protective protein coats that repel the phagocytes. Most dead tissue and foreign particles have no protective coats, which makes them subject to phagocytosis.

When tissue injury occurs multiple substances are released by the injured tissues and cause dramatic secondary changes in the surrounding uninjured tissues of the brain. This entire complex of tissue change is called inflammation.

At times, the macrophages (white blood cells) also further injure the still-living tissue cells. "Walling-off" is the effect of inflammation. "Walling-off" the area of injury from the remaining tissues. This protects the healthy tissue of the brain.

Mitochondria (you have hundreds of these per cell) convert the nutrients from the food you eat into energy that your body uses in order to perform all of the functions it needs to. Alzheimer's is when it identifies that the brain is misusing energy. This abnormality is caused by illness of the mitochondria. When mitochondria turn your food into energy, they produce oxygen free radicals. Molecules that cause dangerous inflammation in the mitochondria themselves as well as in the rest of the cells near the infected area. So we need more antioxidants to clean up this problem.

To understand antioxidants, let's first think about oxygen. Oxygen is necessary for our bodies to function at all. This same oxygen in the form of unstable ions is called free radicals, can oxidize tissues. As a result, oxygen waste products, called lipofuscins, build up in organs such as the heart and brain, leaving brown discoloration on the tissues. These waste products contribute to related aging disease. These spots must be cleaned up by the white blood cells causing more damage to the brain and heart. These brown spots are sign of aging. The older you get, the more prevalent they become.

Imagine an apple, if you slice an apple and leave it out in the air, it will turn brown. The surface of the apple oxidizes, combines with oxygen. This process is similar to what happens when oxygen radicals build up in your body. If you were to take that same apple and sprinkle lemon juice on the slices, they would stay white. The apple does not turn brown because lemon juice is full of vitamin C, which works as an antioxidant. In your body, antioxidants such as vitamins C and E do the same thing by protecting your tissues.

The body can't get rid of free radicals without some help. Antioxidants seek out the roving oxygen radicals and bind to them. Bound together, the free radical and the antioxidant form a bond that the body can then flush out through the kidneys. As long as you have enough antioxidants, free radicals and lipofuscins won't build up in the body.

Oxidation ages your arteries. As you get older, your arteries are more likely to become clogged with fat deposits. These clogs contain high levels of oxidized lipids: fats that have been chemically altered through interaction with high levels of free radicals. Therefore, oxidation plays a significant role in aging of our arteries and effecting your brain. Oxidation affects us in other ways. Oxygen free radicals are an unstable form of oxygen that causes genetic damage. Each cell in your body contains DNA that instructs that cell what to do and when to do it. Oxidation interferes with this process, causing DNA damage. This oxidation is thought to lead to cancer as well as the premature aging of solid tissues. Oxidation can also damage the immune system. Oxidation ages our eyes. It can damage the lenses, promoting cataracts, and the retina. Taken together, vitamins C and E help keep your cardiovascular system healthy by reducing the amount of harmful buildup of plaque on the walls of your arteries. In addition, vitamin C strengthens the immune system, improves both eye and lung function, and helps the body heal. Vitamins C and E, taken in combination, help keep the arteries relaxed and elastic. Take 2,000 mg of vitamin C a day as supplements, in divided doses of no more than 500 mg in any six hours and 400 IU of vitamin E a day, in addition to eating a balanced diet with lots of fresh fruits and vegetables. Vitamin C and vitamin E complement one another. Vitamin C is water soluble, whereas vitamin E is fat -soluble. What does that mean? Cells are made up of two components: The cell membrane and the cell interior. The cell membrane, the outer casing of the cell, consists of lipids, or fats. It is the cell membrane that has the buildup of lipofuscins, those brown spots. Because vitamin E dissolves in fat, it helps prevent oxidant-induced aging in the membrane. In contrast, the inside of the cell consists mostly of water. Because vitamin C dissolves in water, it can enter the center of the cell and collect the free radical. Together, these two vitamins keep oxidants from damaging your cells both inside and out.

People who consume the highest amount of vitamin E are 43% less likely to get Alzheimer's. You can take 400 IU supplement daily if you take it with vitamin C and are not taking statin drugs. In two recently completed randomized studies, vitamin E decreased the progression of Alzheimer's.

If you have elevated blood pressure, it may be because your arteries are constricted, often as a result of cholesterol plaques, and these limit the amount of blood and nutrients that reach a particular area. In the case of the brain, this is what elevates the risk of a stroke or ministrokes throughout the brain. A lack of a healthy blood flow to the brain is one of the main causes of forgetfulness. You can increase the chance of getting Alzheimer's by eating high levels of saturated fats and refined sugar.

Those neurofibrillary tangles associated with Alzheimer's disease contain aluminum. While there is no evidence suggestion that aluminum causes memory problem. It's better to try to avoid it. One way to reduce the aluminum you absorb: Use sea salt instead of table salt, which is processed with aluminum. Other things that contain aluminum include nondairy creamers, antacid, cans, certain cookware, and antiperspirants.

Performing physical activities helps improve long-term memory and brain function. This is logical, as memory and all cognitive functions depend on the health of the arteries. Physical activity helps prevent the arterial aging that contributes to the early onset of Alzheimer's disease, as does playing games that make your mind work.

Early-stage Alzheimer's patients have a new incentive to get moving. A University of Kansas study found that patients who were fit had four times less brain shrinkage (meaning cell death) than those who were out of shape. The benefits of exercise, including changes in growth factors and increased blood vessels and blood flow, may prevent brain cells from dying. Researchers suggest first time exercisers begin with a 15-to 3o-minute walk three times a week.

Does GHRH (growth hormone releasing hormone) improve cognition? When using flexing and massaging your body will produce more GHRH. GHRH is the brain's natural chemical signal for the pituitary gland to secrete growth hormone. Dr. Vitiello and colleagues found that GHRH significantly improved the cognitive function of healthy older men and women, particularly tests of working memory, problem solving and psychomotor processing speed. Their data also showed that GHRH might also be useful in treating individuals with impaired cognitive function, such as those with mild cognitive impairment (MCI) and Alzheimer's disease (AD).

Having MCI is associated with an increased likelihood of continued decline towards a diagnosis of AD. MCI is driven by the assumption that GHRH of older adults with MCI might prevent, or at least delay, cognitive decline towards AD. Delaying progression to AD would be of tremendous benefit to individual patients' quality of life, flexing and massaging will produce GHRH.

The most recent studies on aspirin and aspirin-related drugs show a decrease in the incidence of strokes especially the practically undetectable small-scale, strokes that are often associated with memory loss. Aspirin and chemically similar drugs such as is ibuprofen appear to have this antistroke effect. Best of all, these drugs reduce the incidence of Alzheimer's disease presumably because it helps keep the arteries in the brain young. Aspirin research show a 40% decrease in arterial aging, a major cause of memory loss, for those who take 162 milligrams of aspirin a day. Aspirin helps decrease beta-amyloid from forming in your brain and improves circulation.

Ginkgo Biloba does contain flavonoids and other compounds that are known to scavenge free radicals. Studies indicate possible benefits for people with Alzheimer's disease.

Eating turmeric, which is found in Indian foods lower the incidence of Alzheimer's. India has a relatively low incidence of Alzheimer's.

About five cups of coffee a day protects against cognitive impairment from Alzheimer's. By keeping you alert, caffeine will also help you assimilate knowledge and deposit it in your memory bank efficiently improving the chance that you'll recall it correctly.

Body fitness and weight control greatly reduce vascular disorders that contribute to progression of Alzheimer's disease. This results from maintenance of moderately lower blood pressure and reduced blood cholesterol and low-density lipoprotein (LDL) along with increase high-density lipoprotein (HDL). These changes all work together to reduce the number of brain strokes. There is also accumulating evidence that cerebrovascular disease caused by hypertension (high blood pressure) and atherosclerosis (hardening of the arteries) play a role in Alzheimer's disease. All this can be controlled by your diet, and taking different supplements.

CHAPTER XVIII:
Glycosylation & Multiple Sclerosis

Multiple sclerosis is the most common disabling disorder of the nervous system affecting the young: one in every 1,000 people is affected. MS can cause episodes of blurred or double vision, partial paralysis, clumsiness, and problems with walking.

Glycosylation causes nerve injury. If glucose can't get into a cell, it stays in the blood and causes damage to the nerve cells. When glucose gets inside your nerve cells, it causes big molecules to be built. Not only do these have a problem getting out of the cells easily, but they attract water to those cells, causing them to get bigger. Those big nerve cells get compressed by the tight myelin sheath that surrounds them, eventually damaging those nerves.

Multiple sclerosis is a result of immune system damage to the myelin sheaths that protect nerve fibers. Macrophages (white blood cells which are a type of scavenger cell), remove damaged sections of myelin, so that fibers are exposed and conduct impulses poorly or not at all.

Currently, there is no cure for MS. But I believe that by controlling your sugar intake and having a correct diet this problem can be controlled.

Depending on where glycosylation occurs, it can have a variety of effects on your body. When glucose attaches to a protein (tissues or organs of the body), the altered molecular structure creates different problems throughout the body. In the blood it causes plaque on your arterial walls. In the lens of the eye it causes vision impairment that we call cataract formation. In the skin it causes the collagen to become less elastic.

In your connective tissues when glucose attaches to collagen in your connective tissues, you end up with less elasticity. You need collagen for the smooth functioning of joints. High blood sugar magnifies all aches and pains and can lead to impaired joint movement and eventually arthritis. This can lead to rheumatoid arthritis. This autoimmune form of arthritis develops when the immune system begins to attack body tissues.

Characteristically, many of the small joints are affected in a symmetrical pattern; for example, the hands and feet may be inflamed. The synovial membrane lining an affected joint becomes inflamed. When a tissue becomes inflamed, at least a dozen different products are formed that can cause chemo-taxis toward the inflamed area. The chemotaxis signal can easily move hordes of white blood cells from the capillaries into the inflamed area causing painful deformity. In severe rheumatoid arthritis which leads to phagocytesis, which means cellular ingestion of the offending agent. Joint spaces disappear and the angle at which bone ends meet changes as a result of ligament laxity (looseness). The articular cartilage and the bone ends are eroded. The skin is thin and fragile. These features all restrict movement and cause deformity of the infected area. Again by controlling sugar intake through diet this can be prevented from happening. I believe you can stop this process at an early stage if you restrict your sugar intake and put the disease in prolonged remission.

CHAPTER XIX:

Type 2 Diabetes

What is type 2 diabetes? Type 2 diabetes is far more common than type 1, accounting for about 90 percent of all cases of diabetes mellitus. A combination of abnormalities is responsible for type 2 diabetes. The first is insulin resistance, a condition in which body cells become less responsive to insulin. Development of insulin resistance and impaired glucose metabolism is usually a gradual process, beginning with excess weight gain and obesity. The mechanisms that link obesity with insulin resistance are still uncertain. Studies suggest that there are fewer insulin receptors, especially in the skeletal muscle, liver, and adipose tissue in obese than in lean subjects. Most of the insulin resistances appear to be caused by abnormalities of the signaling pathways that link receptor activation with multiple cellular effects. Impaired insulin signaling appears to be closely related to toxic effects of lipid (fat) accumulation in tissues such as skeletal muscle and liver. Secondary is excess weight gain. Therefore, the body must secrete more insulin to maintain normal metabolism. Insulin resistance, which is very common, doesn't cause type 2 diabetes by itself. The pancreas usually rallies to compensate for the resistance by pumping out more insulin. For most people with insulin resistance, blood sugar levels stay within a normal range. But for some, the insulin-producing cells eventually fail to keep up with the increased demand. Blood sugar levels rise, resulting in type 2 diabetes.

Essentially, type 2 diabetes is a problem of supply and demand. The pancreas supplies too little insulin to keep up with the increased demand that occurs with insulin resistance. For this reason, people with type 2 diabetes can be treated with therapies that decrease insulin demand, with diet and exercise.

One of the most important of all the effects of insulin is to cause most of the glucose absorbed after a meal to be stored almost immediately in the liver in the form of glycogen. Then, between meals, when food is not available and the blood glucose concentration begins to fall, insulin secretion decreases rapidly and the liver glycogen is split back into glucose. This glucose is released back into the blood to keep the glucose concentration from falling too low. When blood glucose is poorly controlled over long periods in type 2 diabetics, blood vessels in multiple tissues throughout the body begin to function abnormally and undergo structural changes that result in inadequate blood supply to the tissues. This in turn leads to increased risk for heart attack, stroke, kidney disease, blindness, and gangrene of the limbs.

While genes, aging, and medications can all cause insulin resistance, being overweight and failing to get enough exercise are major culprits. Of the approximately 1.3 million Americans who will develop type 2 diabetes this year, about 90 percent are overweight or obese. People who are overweight have a body mass index, or BMI, of 25 or more; those who are obese have a BMI of 30 (30% body fat) and above. Weight contributes to insulin resistance. In addition to people who are overweight or sedentary, people over age 65 or who have a family history of type 2 diabetes are at particularly high risk.

There has been a steady increase in the number of younger individuals, some less than 20 years old, with type 2 diabetes. This trend appears to be related mainly to the increasing prevalence of obesity, the most important risk factor for type 2 diabetes in children. Those who have poorly controlled type 2 diabetes throughout childhood are likely to die of heart disease in early adulthood.

Of the more than 18 million people with diabetes in the United States, 90 to 95 percent have type 2 diabetes. The number of adults diagnosed with this disease has increased dramatically-by 65 percent in a little more than a decade.

With increase age, there is a tendency for progressive declines in muscle, leading to "sarcopenia", decreased functional capacity, decreased resting metabolic rate, increased adiposity (fat cells), and increased insulin resistance. Resistance training and aerobic exercise can have a major positive impact for each of these.

The effect of a single bout of aerobic exercise or resistance training on insulin sensitivity last 24–72 hours depending on the duration and intensity of the activity. Because the duration of increased insulin sensitivity is generally not greater than 72 hours. It is recommended that there should not be more than two consecutive days without aerobic physical activity or resistance training.

Lifestyle measures can be taken to assist in the prevention of type 2 diabetes. A person should have a program of weight control, including at least 150 min/week of moderate to vigorous physical activity and a healthful diet with modest energy restriction.

For decades, exercise has been considered a cornerstone of diabetes management, along with diet and medication. However, high-quality evidence on the importance of exercise and fitness in diabetics was lacking until recent years. Recent published documents summarize the most clinically relevant advances related to people with type 2 diabetes and the effect of physical activity/exercise. The publications include greater detail of individual studies, on the prevention of diabetes, as related to the physiology of exercise.

Two randomized trials found that lifestyle intervention including 150 min/week of physical activity and diet-induced weight loss of 5–7% reduced the risk of progression of impaired glucose tolerance (IGT) to type 2 diabetes by 58%. One of the trials found that diet alone, exercise alone, and combined diet and exercise were equally effective in reducing the progression of IGT to diabetes. Therefore, there is consistent evidence that programs of increased physical activity and modest weight loss reduced the incidence of type 2 diabetes in individuals with IGT. The U. S. Surgeon General recommended that most people accumulate 30 min of moderate- intensity activity every days of the week. However, most clinical trials evaluating exercise interventions in people with type 2 diabetes have used a three-times-per-week frequency and many people find it easier to schedule fewer longer sessions rather than five or more weekly shorter sessions. Again, avoid gaps of two or more consecutive days without aerobic physical activity. The effect of resistance exercise training on insulin may last somewhat longer, perhaps because some of it effect are mediated by increases in muscle mass and thereby glucose storage space. Because of the increased evidence for health benefits from resistance training (weight lifting) during the past 10–15 years, the American College of Sports Medicine now recommends that resistance training be included in fitness programs for healthy young and middle-age adults, older adults, and adults with type 2 diabetes.

Moderate exercise is associated with a tenfold increase in fat oxidation (resulting in weight loss). Besides fat mobilization from adipocytes, there is evidence that intramuscular triglycerides represent an important fuel for working muscle. Exercise increases both insulin-independent muscle glucose uptake and insulin sensitivity. Although type 2 diabetic individuals are usually insulin resistant, they are not resistant to the effects of exercise on glucose utilization. It was recently shown that exercise increases the capacity of the liver to consume glucose. The data is consistent displaying that ingestion of glucose immediately after prolonged exercise increased liver glycogen resynthesis. The liver, like muscle, is more insulin sensitive after exercise up to 72 hours.

Exercise has been shown to stimulate insulin in muscles. Regular physical activity leads to an increase in basal and insulin-stimulated pathway activity. Regular physical activities affect insulin signaling. Clinical trials provide strong evidence for the value of physical activity in reducing the incidence of type 2 diabetes. Comparable magnitudes of risk reduction were seen with walking compared with more vigorous activity when total energy expenditure is similar.

It has been hypothesized that an excess accumulation of intramuscular lipid (fats) is associated with insulin resistance in sedentary people. Modest weight loss reduces the incidence of type 2 diabetes.

Type 2 diabetes is associated with reduced muscle mass and muscle strength in older adults. Recent studies using quantitative assessments of muscular function showed that skeletal muscle mass and muscle strength, especially in the lower extremity, is generally lower in adults with type 2 diabetes than in subjects without diabetes. The study was to investigate changes of muscle mass and strength in community dwelling older adults with and without type 2 diabetes. Compared with older adults without diabetes, older adults with type 2 diabetes had greater decreases in leg muscle mass and strength which will result in insulin resistance.

During aging, there is a gradual decrease in the ability to maintain skeletal muscle function and mass. This condition is called "sarcopenia". This process starts at the age of 28 for males, and 33 for females. Fifty percent of the body is muscle mass. As it ages, some of the muscle tissue shrinks and is replaced by fat tissue and fiber. The rate of muscle tissue loss is from three to six percent every ten years and the percentage can be greater if you don't maintain some kind of health care. This is part of the normal aging process. It is the leading cause of insulin resistance. I will explain how this works. A 200 pound person has 100 pounds of muscle mass. If this person losses 6 percent of muscle by the age of 38; he will have lost 6 pounds of muscle mass. At the age of 68 this person will have lost 24 pounds of muscle mass. This is 24 percent of this person muscle mass resulting in insulin resistance. The human body has 100 trillion cells, and about 50 trillion are muscle cells. Each cell contains mitochondria. Mitochondria are present in all areas of each cell's cytoplasm, but the total number per cell varies from less than a hundred up to several thousand, depending on the amount of energy (this energy is made by the mitochondria) required by the cell. The mitochondria are concentrated in those portions of the cell that are responsible for the major share of its energy metabolism (like muscle cells). More than 95 percent of this ATP (energy) is formed in the mitochondria, which accounts for the mitochondria being called the "power houses" of the cell.

Each muscle cell has 2,000 mitochondria. The body has 50 trillion muscle cells x 2,000 mitochondria which equals 100,000 trillion mitochondria. When your body losses one percent of its muscle mass it will loss 100 trillion mitochondria, which will lead to insulin resistance. The body produces the same amount of fuel, but it doesn't need this amount because it has less muscle mass and mitochondria's to produce energy (Fuel – Muscle Mass = Insulin Resistance). This results in the cells becoming insulin resistance.

When people with type 2 diabetes exercise they make the cell use more fuel for energy. This results in the cell becoming insulin sensitive for 24 to 72 hours depending on the type and length of exercise. With flexing and massaging you will regain all your muscle mass and mitochondria's which will protect you from type 2 diabetes.

CHAPTER XX:

Diet

More than 9,000 scientific studies have proven beyond doubt—food (diet) is your best medicine! By using Mother Nature's most delicious foods to lose weight, prevent cancer, reverse heart disease, prevent neurological disorders, cleanse your arteries, and lower your cholesterol, look and feel years younger, a person can dramatically increase their longevity. Diet has an effect on arthritis pain. Inflammation is a root problem in arthritis, and it is often directly responsible for joint pain and tissue damage. Your food choices can either increase or decrease inflammation.

The first rule is to avoid refined, processed, and manufactured foods, most of which contain pro-inflammatory fats, carbohydrates, and additives. Omega-6 fatty acids intensify inflammation, and most people eat too much of them; a major source is refined soybean oil, a cheap ingredient in many processed foods such as cookies, crackers, and snacks. Another culprit is high-fructose corn syrup, the ubiquitous sweetener. It is a quickly digested carbohydrate that disturbs metabolism in many people and favors production of inflammation-promoting substances in the body.

When preparing your food, use good quality extra-virgin olive oil. Its unique antioxidant helps protect all tissues from inflammatory damage. Be sure also to increase consumption of anti-inflammatory omega-3 fatty acids by eating oily fish at least three times a week. Take two to three grams of supplemental fish oil, which is recommend to most people, certainly those with arthritis.

Learn to distinguish good carbs from bad carbs by understanding glycemic load. This is the measure of how carbohydrate foods affect blood sugar. Minimizing spikes in blood sugar by reducing glycemic load of meals helps contain inflammation. Replace high-glycemic-load foods (simple carbohydrates), such as those made with flour and sugar, with foods that have lower glycemic loads (complex carbohydrates), such as whole or cracked grains, sweet potatoes, winter squashes, and beans. Moderate portions of pasta are better than most breads and potatoes.

Reduce consumption of animal protein, especially red meat and dark chicken, which contain a pro-inflammatory amino acid. Eat plenty of fruits and vegetables that cover the color spectrum. The pigments in these foods have health-protective effects. Try to find ways to consume ginger and turmeric in any forms; both spices have powerful anti-inflammatory effects. Add a teaspoon of powdered turmeric to soups, stews, and other dishes.

The miracle diet protects your heart and prevents a slew of diseases with this tasty, traditional way of eating. Scientist have long touted the benefits of the diet for heart health. But there's more and more evidence that the diet can keep you healthy in other ways too. Diet cuts the risk of death from all causes by 20 percent.

When you have breakfast you need to choose complex carbs. Making your daily cereal, bread or baked good the whole-grain kind is great for your heart. And since whole wheat and oats retain their fiber-rich bran and germ, they safeguard against the insulin surges that refined carbohydrates cause. The result: In a Harvard study of 43,000 men, those who ate the most wholegrain foods cut their diabetes risk in half.

Lunch should lean toward leafy greens to lower the cardiovascular risk. The great part is the more greens you eat, the lower your risk gets. They are also major cancer fighters, by more than 40 percent. The folate found in spinach, endive, and romaine can help your brain age gracefully. Diets high in the B vitamin protected 50 to 85 years old subjects against cognitive declines, in a study at Tufts University.

At dinner individuals need to eat more fish. Omega-3 fats in seafood are the newest nutrition all-stars. They protect against heart disease, and recent research has also linked them to lower rates of both depression and Alzheimer's disease. Eating far more fish than red meat additionally earns you an anticancer edge: Colorectal cancer risk was 30 percent lower in people who ate the most seafood. Among people who ate the most red meat, the risk increased by more than one third as reported in the Journal of the Nation Cancer Institute. Eating the right amounts of omega-3 fats helps to unlock stored body fat so that you can use it better as energy. Omega-3 fat balances your body's ratio of insulin to glucagon. When you eat sugary foods, your body secretes the hormone insulin to remove the excess sugar from your body. When you eat excessively sugary meals, your body releases too much insulin, blocking the critical pancreatic hormone glucagon from operating effectively within your body. Glucagon is a key hormone that enables your body to burn its stores of body fat. A diet rich in omega-3 fats helps balance your insulin levels so that glucagon can be released to unlock your body's fat-storage banks and begin converting unwanted body fat into energy. Omega-3 fats boost your body's metabolic rate, which in turn helps you burn more body fat.

Though any fat can help satisfy your appetite or even release stored body fat, omega fats and particularly the omega-3's, offer a number of uniquely wonderful benefits. They cannot ever be converted into the "bad" saturated fats. This is important because excessive intake of saturated fat is closely linked to obesity, cancer, heart disease, stroke, and premature death. Hundreds of research studies show that omega-3 fats can actually help prevent all of these things, plus certain types of diabetes. In women, omega fats have been shown to help ease premenstrual syndrome and postmenopausal discomforts. In men, omega-3 fats have been shown to improve sex drive.

A study found that supplementing the diet with omega-3 fats changed the composition of joint cartilage, reducing the pain and inflammation associated with various types of arthritis. Another study found that patients who took omega-3 supplements were able to completely stop taking their anti-inflammatory painkillers for arthritic disease.

A study found that people who eat more omega-3 fats on a daily basis experience a lower risk of prostate cancer and prostate inflammation. Numerous other studies have shown a decreased risk for other types of cancers as well.

A study found that supplementing with omega-3 fats reduced some of the intestinal inflammation associated with Crohn's disease. Many other studies have shown that diets high in omega-3 fats reduce all sorts of gastrointestinal problems, from chronic diarrhea to chronic constipation.

Research strongly shows that increasing the omega fats in your diet while simultaneously decreasing the saturated and trans fats can boost immunity, regulate blood sugar, prevent diabetes, reduce heart disease and stroke, treat asthma, lift depression, and prevent Alzheimer's disease. You should swap spices for salt. Herbs such as sage and oregano help battle insulin resistance, a blunting of the body's ability to balance blood sugar that can raise risks of heart disease and stroke by 28 and 64 percent, respectively. In a USDA experiment, researchers found that sage and oregano doubled insulin activity, while turmeric and cloves tripled it. That's good news for anyone trying to keep blood sugar stable. In other words, for anyone who wants to protect their health cinnamon proved the top performer and in a subsequent study, diabetics who ate one gram of cinnamon (less than half a teaspoon) per day for 40 days lowered their fasting blood sugar by 18 percent and their LDL by 7 percent.

A dessert option is to enjoy different kinds of fruit. Treats such as figs and dates are tops in the amount of fiber and potassium. Potassium is a mineral that plays a key role in blood pressure control. Since their antioxidant content is up to 50 times higher than that of other fruit, they are an absolute feast for the eyes: Eating three or more servings of high antioxidant fruit a day lowers the risk of sight-robbing age-related maculopathy by 36 percent in people 50 and up, a Harvard study showed.

When it is snack time individuals should nibble on nuts. Almonds and pistachios have impressive cholesterol-lowering powers: In separate studies at the University of Toronto and Penn State, eating two handfuls a day dropped subjects' evil LDL by 9.4 and 11.6 percent, respectively. Nuts' satisfying nature protects against added pounds. People who ate nuts at least twice a week were 31 percent less likely to gain weight than those who rarely or never ate them.

Protein is your body's building material. You need to eat protein to provide your body with the materials it needs to build, repair, and maintain your lean muscle tissue. Over half of your body weight is made up of protein. When you don't eat enough protein, your body actually starts to break down and recycle existing body protein (such as lean muscle) to supply your body with the amino acids that your diet is lacking. When this protein breakdown occurs, you sacrifice muscle (your fat-burning machine) and your metabolism slows down. As a result, you burn less body fat.

Unfortunately, protein is a "dirty" source of fuel because it contains nitrogen. Instead of producing just carbon dioxide and water, protein produces nitrogenous residues, which are toxic. Your body must pump a lot of water into the urinary tract to flush the toxic nitrogen out. Much of the weight loss from high-protein diets is simply water loss. While this is going on, you're also losing minerals from your body, including calcium from your bones.

One thing you can be sure of is that processed meats contain nitrates to convey flavor, give meats their blood-red color, and resist the development of botulism spores. Nitrates can convert to nitrites, which have been studied for decades in public and private settings and found to cause cancer and tumors in test animals.

Our meat and dairy supply is loaded with growth hormones. These hormones are given to the animals to speed growth in order to increase production and profits. When you consume meat and dairy you are giving yourself massive amounts of growth hormone. This leads to obesity, cancer, and is one the reasons why children today are maturing earlier.

Besides getting protein in the right amounts, you also want to focus on the right types. Some types of protein-especially the type found in animal products-contain a high amount of saturated fat, which can not only hinder your weight-loss efforts but also destroy your health. Focus on high-quality protein sources like fish, skinless white-meat chicken, turkey meat, soy products, egg whites, legumes, and beans.

Soybeans are a quality protein source that is naturally low in saturated fat. If you're a vegetarian, eating soy is the best way to ensure that you consume all of the amino acids you need. Even if you're not a vegetarian, I recommend adding soy to your diet because it has been shown to reduce heart disease, cancer, osteoporosis, menopausal symptoms, and more.

When you have a hankering for red meat, go ahead and have it, but choose lean sirloin or round cuts, eat a small portion, and trim off any visible fat. Limit your red meat consumption to once a week or less. Beef comes marbled with nonessential fat that is mostly saturated. It is the worst animal fat in terms of chemical composition, containing 51 percent saturated fatty acids. In comparison, pig lard, still very bad, has 41 percent saturated fatty acids.

WATER

The typical person needs eight 8-ounce glasses of water a day. Your body needs water for everything from maintaining blood volume to skin health to toxin release. Without it, your energy level plummets, and you get headaches. That's because the electrical and chemical signals in your brain work on water. Dehydration also lowers your blood volume, making your heart pump harder to move blood throughout your body.

Water takes up room in your stomach, making you feel full. That means you eat less and feel full. Of all the ways you can get fluid into your body, drinking water is the best because it has no calories. Drinking more water and fewer liquid calories will suppress your hunger, lower your calorie intake, cleanse your body, and give you more energy.

THE PLAN

Despite a multibillion-dollar diet industry, we're overweight and nothing we do seems to work. America is getting more and more obese. Obesity in children and adults in the United States is rapidly increasing, rising by more than 30 percent over the past decade. Approximately 64 percent of adults in the United States are overweight, and nearly 33 percent of adults are obese. Obesity is usually defined as 25 percent or greater total body fat in men and 35 percent or greater in women.

Childhood over nutrition is the cause of obesity in children. The rate of formation of new fat cells is especially rapid in the first few years of life, and the greater the rate of fat storage, the greater the number of fat cells. The number of fat cells in obese children is often as much as three times that in normal children. It has been suggested that over nutrition of children especially in infancy and during the later years of childhood can lead to a lifetime of obesity. It's one of the nation's biggest health problems and it's growing by the day. The Center for Disease Control and Prevention now estimate that approximately 19 percent of adolescents (ages 12–19) are considered overweight. These numbers have nearly tripled among children and quadrupled among adolescents during the last 25 years. Researchers predict that nearly half the children in North America will be overweight by 2010, and data indicates that 80 percent of these children will likely be overweight as adults, placing them at a higher risk of developing health problems like high cholesterol, hypertension and diabetes. IT IS UP TO THE PARENTS TO CONTROL THE DAILY INTAKE OF FOOD OF THE INFANT AT BIRTH TO REDUCE THE NUMBER OF FAT CELLS BEING FORMED TO CONTROL THE PROBLEM OF OBESITY!!!!! Nearly 25 percent of American kids are either overweight or obese.

Some scientists believe that today's generation of overweight children will have shorter life spans than their parents. Globally it is estimated that 250 million people worldwide are obese. If current trends continue obesity will overtake smoking as the primary cause of preventable death. A startling study showed that obese children and teens have arteries that look like those of an average 45-year-old. Kids with high cholesterol showed the same dismal changes. "Obesity in adolescents is a time bomb," say Juan Alejos, MD, a pediatric cardiologist. "By 2035 there will be 100,000 extra cases of adult heart disease because of obesity in today's children."

You may have heard that obesity is increasingly being diagnosed in young people in America. Take the time to ask some difficult questions about your child's health habits: Does your child eat a healthy diet? Is he or she active enough? Is he or she overweight? Parents need to pay attention to the habits their children are learning and make sure they are healthy habits. Healthy habits matter. Being overweight and inactive are risk factors. Lifestyle changes can make a difference.

All children need to eat a healthier diet. The first thing is cutting out soda and juice because kids are drinking far too many calories a day. Serve fruits and vegetables, watch portion sizes, set regular eating times, avoid skipping meals, and have meals sitting down at a table.

Kids should get at least 60 minutes of activity a day. It does not need to be formal exercise. Playing on the playground counts. You can help boost activity levels by reducing TV and computer time. To help keep kids active, you can: Assign active chores, have kids walk or ride their bikes to school, and find a physical activity the whole family enjoys.

Families have an important role to play. Lifestyle changes have to be family changes. Success comes when the family works together to have a positive impact on their child health.

Approximately three hundred thousand American will die prematurely from obesity this year. Obesity often attributed to high blood pressure. With high blood pressure, the heart must work harder to push blood through the arteries. This never-ending workout causes the heart to grow. An enlarged heart can place undue strain on the muscle and result in sudden cardiac arrest.

Blood circulation needs help to get the venous blood back up to the heart from the legs. Under normal conditions, assistance comes from the muscles in the legs. They help pump blood towards the heart by squeezing the deep veins in the legs. But when you're obese, you don't have enough muscle to do this, so blood pools in the veins, and clots may form. The clot sometimes breaks free and floats into the lungs, and may cause sudden death.

Excessive weight takes a toll on the body and can take up to twenty years off your life. It's very difficult for people who are obese to be completely healthy. They run a risk of coronary heart disease, stroke, high blood pressure, cancer, diabetes, gout, arthritis, gallstones, infertility, injuries due to falls, and childbirth complications, compare to people of normal weight.

There are diseases like sleep apnea and fatty liver disease. Sleep apnea occurs when you stop breathing momentarily many times throughout the night because your airways become blocked when muscles in your throat relax. Anatomical problems such as fat around the pharynx contribute to the problem. Obesity is a risk factor for sleep apnea, and 30 percent of people with a BMI over 30 (30 percent body fat) will have obstructive sleep apnea. Sleep apnea can increase the risk of heart attack, stroke, and high blood pressure. Many times you don't know you have it unless your bedmate notices it or hears you snoring loudly. People with this disorder stop breathing for 10 to 30 seconds or more at a stretch during sleep, up to 400 times each night. The loss of oxygen kills off brain cells in regions that regulate blood pressure. That can trigger hypertension or wide swings in blood pressure, which can lead to a stiffening of blood vessels. Weight loss is one of the simpler treatments for sleep apnea.

More and more obese people are turning up with fatty liver disease, a buildup of fat in the liver cells. Fat cells in the belly do more damage because they release fatty acids and other substances that travel directly to the liver. This can cause liver inflammation and, sometimes, the formation of fibrous tissue. This can lead to either cirrhosis or liver cancer. A man with a waist bigger than about 40 inches is twice as likely to die prematurely as a man whose waist is less than about 34 inches, a study of more than 350,000 people found last year. For women, a waist of more than 35 inches is a red flag.

When you lose weight-even as little as 10 to 15 percent of your weight-these problems get better. This suggests that obesity plays a big role in their development.

Obesity is the results from greater energy intake than energy expenditure. When greater quantities of energy (in the form of food) enter the body than are expended, the body weight increases, and most of the excess energy is stored as fat. Excessive obesity is caused by energy intake in excess of energy output. For each 9.3 Calories of excess energy that enter the body approximately 1 gram of fat is stored (28 grams equal one ounce and 16 ounces equal one pound). Recent studies have shown that the development of obesity in adults is accompanied by increased numbers, as well as increased size, of adipocytes (fat cell). An extremely obese person may have as many as four times as many adipocytes, each containing twice as much lipid, as a lean person. The rapid increase of obesity in the past 20 to 30 years emphasized the important role of lifestyle and environmental factors, because genetic changes could not have occurred so rapidly.

Within the past few years, science has linked our ravenous appetites to hormones. Among the hormones that fuel these urges are ghrelin and leptin. Ghrelin is produced mostly by cells in the stomach lining. Its job is to make you feel hungry by affecting the hypothalamus, which governs metabolism. Ghrelin levels rise in dieters who lose weight and then try to keep it off. It's almost as if their bodies are trying to regain the lost fat. This is one reason why it's hard to lose weight and maintain the loss.

Leptin turns your appetite off and is made by fat cells. Low leptin levels increase your appetite and signal your body to store more fat. High leptin levels relay the opposite signal. Many obese people have developed a resistance to the appetite-suppressing effects of leptin and never feel satisfied, no matter how much they eat. Your body uses these hormones to help you stay at your weight and keep you from losing fat-which is another reason why dieting can be so difficult.

Lack of sleep promotes obesity by messing with these hunger hormones. If you skimp on sleep, ghrelin levels rise, making you hungry, and leptin levels dip, which signals a need for calories.

For someone hugely overweight people, minor surgery becomes major surgery and infinitely more risky. Some of these increased risks include difficulty with intubation and anesthesia, poor wound healing, increased risk of infection, and post surgical blood clots, not to mention the technical difficulties the surgeon often encounters due to the fatty tissue itself.

Approximately three hundred thousand Americans will die prematurely from obesity this year, and millions more will know its agony. Anyone who puts on pounds year after year is at risk for becoming overweight, obese, or even morbidly obese.

Regular physical activity and physical training are known to increase muscle mass and decrease body fat mass, whereas inadequate physical activity is typically associated with decreased muscle mass and increased adiposity (fat cells). For example, studies have shown a close association between sedentary behaviors, such as prolonged television watching, and obesity.

About 25 to 30 percent of the energy used each day by the average person goes into muscular activity, and in a laborer, as much as 60 to 70 percent is used in this way. In obese people, increased physical activity usually increases energy expenditure more than food intake resulting in significant weight loss. Even a single episode of strenuous exercise may increase basal energy expenditure for several hours after the physical activity is stopped. Because muscular activity is by far the most important means by which energy is expended in the body, increased physical activity is often an effective means of reducing fat stored. To obtain an increase in muscle mass, flexing and massaging muscles, will burn more energy.

Treatment of obesity depends on decreasing energy input below energy expenditure and creating a sustained negative energy balance until the desire weight loss is achieved. This means either reducing energy intake or increasing energy expenditure. The current National Institutes of Health guidelines recommend a decrease in caloric intake of 500 kilocalories per day for overweight and moderately obese person (25 to 35 percent body fat) to achieve a weight loss of approximately 1 pound each week. A more aggressive energy deficit of 500 to 1000 kilocalories per day is recommended for person with a greater than 35 percent body fat to loss approximately 2 pound per week. For most people attempting to lose weight, increasing physical activity is an important component of successful long-term weight loss. The most dramatic increase that occurs in fat utilization is that observed during heavy exercise. This causes rapid breakdown of triglycerides from the fat cells. The triglycerides concentrations in the blood of an exercising person rise as much as eightfold, and are used by the muscles for energy is increased. Exercise promotes weight loss by helping you to burn more calories than you take in.

One of the ways that an individualized exercise plan is broken down is by the number of calories they burn. Calories are merely a measure of energy. The number of calories in a food indicates how much energy it will give you; the number of calories burned by an activity indicates how much energy is used when you do that activity.

Remember, even if you were very athletic earlier in your life, getting started again can be a humbling-and even dangerous-experience if you don't take proper precautions. So don't push yourself, start slow and work gradually toward your goals. It is very important for you to check with your personal physician before beginning any new exercise program. This is doubly important if you're at personal risk for coronary heart disease, or someone who's overweight or severely out of shape. You and your doctor, or personal trainer must design an exercise program for you that will minimize your risk of event.

Exercise will be easier if you move into it gradually. If you start with a 10-minute walk every day and increase it by 5 minutes every week, you'll be walking a total of 60 minutes in 10 weeks. Easing into exercise will help reduce the chance of joint, bone, and muscle injury.

Once you're ready to begin an exercise program, your next step is to figure out the kinds of things you like to do. If you can bring the play back into your exercise life, then you'll reduce boredom and increase your enjoyment, and that means you'll be more likely to do it.

If you're just starting an exercise program or if you have physical limitations, you'll probably want to stick with low-impact exercise, like swimming and walking.

Exercise also has a profound effect on the way your body's metabolism works. Working out actually makes your body more efficient. When it comes to improving your metabolic profile through exercise is an enzyme called lipoprotein lipase, or LPL. LPL is like a furry lining attached to the inside of your arteries. As the blood passes through, it rubs up against that hairy lining, and a number of processes occur. This enzyme determines how fast your body chews up triglycerides. If the LPL enzyme is working well and efficiently, your body is chewing up fats in the bloodstream very quickly. Exercise sends a message to increase production of LPL. Because your body anticipates the need for more energy, which it gets from triglycerides, it creates more LPL to help it metabolize the triglycerides. The more LPL you produce, the faster you pull fats from your bloodstream. LPL production can be generated for up to 23 hours after exercise. This is one important reason why it makes sense for people who are trying to control high triglycerides to work out every day. Being active-either through physical activity or through a formal exercise program-is an essential component for weight-loss. When you're active, your body uses energy (calories) to work, helping to burn the calories you take in with the food you eat. Whatever activity you choose, the key is to commit to doing it regularly. Aim for 30 to 60 minutes of moderately intensive physical activity most days of the week.

The below chart displays the estimated number of calories burned while performing a variety of exercises for one hour. Calorie expenditure varies widely depending on the exercise, intensity level and individual.

Individuals Weight	140	180	220
Aerobic, high impact	511	637	763
Aerobic, low impact	364	455	545
Aerobic water	292	364	436
Bicycling, less 10 mph	292	364	436
Dancing	219	273	327
Golf, carrying clubs	329	410	491
Hiking	438	546	654
Jogging, 5 mph	584	728	872
Rope jumping	511	637	763
Running, 8 mph	986	1,229	1,472
Rowing, stationary	511	637	763
Swimming laps	511	637	763
Stair treadmill	657	819	986
Walking, 2 mph	188	228	273
Walking, 3.5 mph	277	346	481
Weight lifting	219	273	327

Exercise is important: Studies show that it staves off heart trouble, lowers blood pressure, normalizes blood sugar, strengthens bone health, improves depression and anxiety, and keeps your brain up to par as you age, among many other benefits. Extensive research has demonstrated that people who exercise tend to live longer. Try to find ways of making exercise an unavoidable part of your everyday life, so at work take the stairs. When running errands, pick the farthest parking space out. There are plenty of ways to work exercise into your life: Play with your kids, garden and do yard work, walk briskly around the mall when you're shopping, walk your dog, clean your house, cook more meals at home, or go dancing. What you do will depend on your physical condition and what you most enjoy doing, but most people can get started with some simple shifts in these lifestyle activities or a walking program.

The Sienkiewicz diet: The major foods on which the body lives can be classified as carbohydrates, fats, and proteins. All the energy foods can be oxidized in the cells, and during these process large amounts of energy are released. The major function is energy is required for muscle activity. The amount of energy of a food is expressed in terms of calories.

The final products of carbohydrate digestion are almost entirely glucose. When glucose is not immediately required for energy, the extra glucose that continually enters the cells is either stored as glycogen or converted into fat. Glucose is preferentially store as glycogen until the cells have stored as much glycogen as they can-an amount sufficient to supply the energy needs of the body for only 12 to 24 hours.

When the glycogen-storing cells (primarily liver and muscle cells) approach saturation with glycogen, the additional glucose is converted into fat in liver and fat cells and is stored as fat in the fat cells, causing an increase in weight. Several chemical compounds in food and in the body are classified as lipids (fats). They include (1) neutral fat, also known as triglycerides; (2) phospholipids; and (3) cholesterol. The triglycerides are used in the body mainly to provide energy for the different metabolic processes, a function they share almost equally with the carbohydrates.

Almost all the fats in the diet are absorbed from the intestines into the intestinal lymph. They are transported upward through the thoracic duct and emptied into the circulating venous blood at the juncture of the jugular and subclavian veins.

Large quantities of fat are stored in two major tissues of the body, the adipose tissue and the liver. The major function of adipose tissue is storage of triglycerides until they are needed to provide energy elsewhere in the body. The fat cells (adipocytes) of adipose tissue are stored almost pure triglycerides in quantities as great as 80 to 95 per cent of the entire cell volume. Triglycerides inside the fat cells are generally in a liquid form only liquid fat can be hydrolyzed and transported from the cells.

Large quantities of triglycerides appear in the liver in which fat instead of carbohydrates is being used for energy. In these conditions, large quantities of triglycerides are mobilized from the adipose tissue, transported in the blood to the liver, where the initial stages of much of fat degradation begin. Under normal physiologic conditions, the total amount of triglycerides in the liver is determined to a great extent by the overall rate at which lipids are being used for energy.

About 40 per cent of the calories in a typical American diet are derived from fats which are almost equal to the calories derived from carbohydrates. The use of fats by the body for energy is as important as the use of carbohydrates. When to many carbohydrates are ingested with each meal they are converted into triglycerides, then stored and used later in the form of fatty acids released from the triglycerides for energy. When carbohydrates are not used for energy, almost all the energy of the body must come from metabolism of fats. The unavailability of carbohydrates automatically increases the rate of removal of fatty acids from adipose tissues. By decreasing the intake of carbohydrates and fats, and using energy from fat cells will result in weight loss.

The ability of the different cells of the body to store carbohydrates in the form of glycogen is generally slight; a maximum of only a few hundred grams of glycogen can be stored in the liver, the skeletal muscles, and all other tissues of the body put together. In contrast, many kilograms of fat can be stored. Fat synthesis provides a means by which the energy of excess ingested carbohydrates, fats, and proteins can be stored for later use. The average person has almost 150 times as much energy stored in the form of fat as stored in the form of carbohydrate. Each gram of fat contains almost two and a half times the calories of energy contained by each gram of glycogen. For a given weight gain, a person can store several times as much energy in the form of fat as in the form of carbohydrate. When people have more proteins in their diet than their tissues can use as proteins, a large share of the excess is stored as fat. An increase in the amount of cholesterol ingested each day increases the plasma concentration slightly. Plasma cholesterol concentration usually is not changed upward or downward more than + or − 15 per cent by altering the amount of cholesterol in the diet, although the response of individuals differs markedly.

A highly saturated fat diet increases blood cholesterol concentration 15 to 25 per cent. This result from increased fat deposition in the liver. To decrease the blood cholesterol concentration, it is usually just as important, if not more important, to maintain a diet low in saturated fat as to maintain a diet low in cholesterol.

Ingestion of fat containing highly unsaturated fatty acids (omega-3) usually depresses the blood cholesterol concentration a slight to moderate amount. The mechanism of this effect is unknown, despite the fact that this observation is the basis of much present-day dietary strategy.

Intake of carbohydrates, fats, and proteins provides energy that can be used to perform various body functions or stored for later use. Stability of body weight and composition over long periods requires that a person's energy intake and energy expenditure be balanced. When a person is overfed and energy intake persistently exceeds expenditure, most of the excess energy is stored as fat and body weight increases; loss of body mass occurs when energy intake is insufficient to meet the body's metabolic needs. Because different foods contain different proportions of proteins, carbohydrates, fats, minerals, and vitamins, appropriate balances must also be maintained among these constituents so that all segments of the body's metabolic systems can be supplied with these materials. I'll discusses the mechanisms by which food intake is regulated in accordance with the body's metabolic needs and some of the problems of maintaining balance among the different types of foods.

The energy from each gram of carbohydrate is 4.1 Calories, and that liberated from fat is 9.3 Calories. The average energy from protein for each gram is 4.35 Calories. Average American receives about 15 per cent of their energy from protein, 40 per cent from fat, and 45 percent from carbohydrate.

When food is high in fat you consume a much higher number of calories. While it's true that some fat is needed in the diet, fat is for the most part provides little in the way of vitamins and minerals. Many of these empty calories come from meat, cheese, eggs, milk, and nuts.

The goal then, for those who are trying to lose or maintain their weight, must be to minimize their fat intake and to avoid foods that derive the majority of their calories from fat.

Cheddar cheese gets 70 percent of its calories from fat, while cottage cheese gets 30 percent. Hot dogs and bologna get 90 percent of their calories from fat. Skinless white chicken gets 20 percent. Peanuts and salad dressing can get up to 90 percent of their calories from fat. Light yogurt can be as little as 5 percent.

Selecting fish, white chicken without the skin, low- and non-fat dairy products, and almonds over peanuts are all ways to reduce fat intake. Use sparingly, or purchase non-fat/low-fat versions of, butter, oils, mayonnaise, and salad dressings. Be sure to use cooking techniques that do not add additional fats to your meals.

Always refer to nutritional labels when buying foods. A quick label glance will tell you how many grams of fat a food item contains, how many calories are in one serving and what percentage of those calories are coming from fat. Successfully minimizing your fat intake can help you eat healthier, feel better and look trimmer.

Twenty to thirty grams of the body proteins are degraded and used to produce other body chemicals daily. Therefore, all cells must continue to form new proteins to take the place of those that are being destroyed, and a supply of protein is needed in the diet for this purpose. An average person can maintain normal stores of protein, provided the daily intake is above 30 to 50 grams.

Treatment of a diet to lose weight depends on decreasing energy input below energy expenditure and creating a sustained negative energy balance until the desired weight loss is achieved. This means either reducing energy intake or increasing energy expenditure with exercise for best result doing both of these is the correct means of achieving weight loss.

Now we must figure out how many calories we need each day to lose weight. We all burn calories just by existing. If you never got out of bed at all, you still burn a certain number of calories. This is called your basal metabolic rate (BMR). You need that number of calories simply to survive. You can figure out your own BMR using the Harris-Benedict Equations.

Men
66
+(13.7 x weight in kilograms)
+(5 X height in centimeters)
−(6.8 x age in years)

BMR=
Women
655
+(9.6 x weight in kilograms)
+(1.8 x height in centimeters)
−(4.7 x age in years)

BMR=

Get a calculator, and your weight in kilograms is your weight in pounds divided by 2.2 So if you weigh 180 pounds, divide that number by 2.2 to get 81.8 kilograms. Your height in centimeters is your height in inches multiplied by 2.54 If you're 5'8" tall, you're 68 inches. 68 inches multiplied by 2.54 is 172.72 centimeters. A 5'8" man is 173 centimeters tall. The BMR for a 64-year man, who is 5'8" tall and 180 pounds would be:

BMR = 66 + (13.7 x 81.8)+(5 x 173) − (6.8 x 64) = 1,617 calories. This provides you with a very good starting point. Nobody stays in bed all day-even if your daily exercise isn't more than light activity; you're burning more than your BMR as soon as you get out of bed.

This activity multiplier will help you to discover approximately how many calories you're actually burning every day.

Little or no exercise, desk job = BMR x 1.2

Exercise 1 to 3 days a week = BMR x 1.375

Exercise 6 or 7 days a week = BMR x 1.55

Hard exercise 6 or 7 days a week = BMR x 1.725

Hard daily exercise and hard physical job = BMR x 1.9

If you've done your own calculations, you'll know how many calories you're burning every day. You must run a calorie deficit to lose weight. It's like balancing a budget. If you make more calories than you burn, your weight will increase. If you burn more calories than you take in, you will lose weight.

Calories required to survive + extra calories= FAT!

The rule for losing weight is simple: Eat fewer calories than you burn. So it's a good idea to get familiar with the calorie count of foods. Just a couple of days of using a calorie-counting book, calculating the calories you consume, and writing them down can really help. You don't have to do this forever, just long enough to get a feel for it. You should burn 500 calories less than your BMR to lose weight (BMR-500 calories = weight loss). IF you burn 500 calories; this equals 53 grams of fat loss or 1.9 ounces (500 divided by 9.4 = 53 grams divided by 28 = 1.9 ounces). When carbohydrates are not used for energy almost all the energy of the body must come from metabolism of fats. The unavailability of carbohydrates automatically increases the rate of removal of fatty acids from adipose tissues (fat cells). By decreasing the intake of carbohydrates and fats, and using energy from fat cells will result in weight loss.

So the plan is to eat complex carbohydrates (fruits, vegetables, and whole grains) and curtail the intake of simple carbohydrates. You must not eat anything with white flour and white sugar. White bread and French fries are very high in simple carbohydrates. One finding was that certain starches such as white bread and white potatoes increase blood sugar levels faster than table sugar does. Soda pop and juices with high sugar content must not be consumed (drink water). Refined carbs cause rapid changes in blood sugar levels, stimulate further hunger, thereby encouraging overeating and obesity.

The complex carbohydrates are lower in carbohydrates and contain some proteins. Complex carbohydrates are absorbed into the bloodstream more slowly, and release energy slowly into the system.

Now you must eliminate the intake of saturated fats in your diet. Foods like beef, pork, lamb, dark chicken, whole-milk cheese, ice cream, and whole milk. Replace these with unsaturated fats. Foods like fish, skinless chicken, and turkey (white meat).

By eating the correct number of calories: Eating complex carbohydrates and unsaturated fat. You will start getting your energy from your fat cells and this spells weight loss.

The perfect diet (Sienkiewicz) is to become choosy about the food you eat-not just for a couple of weeks or months but for the rest of your life. The perfect diet is not really a diet at all, but a way of eating you can live with every day.

Starvation is the depletion of food stores in the body tissues. When my mother went to a care facility. I watched her body deteriorate into skin and bones. It was very sad and hard to watch. After her death I learned how this process worked. I will explain what happened to create this deterioration and how to prevent this from happening to you. Even though the tissues preferentially use carbohydrate for energy over both fat and protein, the quantity of carbohydrate normally stored in the entire body is only a few hundred grams. It can supply the energy required for body function for perhaps half a day. Therefore, except for the first few hours of starvation, the major effects are progressive depletion of tissue fat and protein. Because fat is the prime source of energy (100 times fat energy is stored in the normal person as carbohydrate energy), the rate of fat depletion continues until most of the stored fat in the body is gone. Protein undergoes three phases of depletion; rapid depletion at first, then greatly slowed depletion, and finally rapid depletion again shortly before death.

There finally comes a time when the fat stores are depleted, and the only remaining source of energy is protein. At that time, the protein stores (muscle mass) once again enters a stage of rapid depletion. Because proteins are also essential for the maintenance of cellular function, death ordinarily ensues when the proteins of the body have been depleted to about half their normal level. To prevent this from happening you must have a large intake of both simple and complex carbohydrates. The care facility didn't want my mother eating simple carbohydrate because it would interfere with her diet;

resulting in starvation (she really enjoyed eating these types of foods, candy, chips, bread, ect). She never liked the food in the care facility and this was a very expensive care facility. By using flexing and massaging (regaining your muscle mass), and eating simple and complex carbohydrate you have a good chance of leaving the rest home, and returning home. Barring any other medical conditions that would prevent your release.

I would like to point out one other problem then you are in a care facility. Lying motionless in bed for many days can lead to the development of bedsores (muscle breakdown). When you lie stationary for an extended period of time, your skeletal muscles can begin to physically deteriorate. As these muscles break down, they release a protein called myoglobin that does damage to the kidneys. Every day the patient should try to walk or set in a chair to relieve the pressure on these muscles.

CHAPTER XXI:

Sports Physiology

There are few stresses to which the body is exposed that even nearly approach the extreme stresses of heavy exercise. In fact, if some of the extremes of exercise were continued for even moderately prolonged periods, they might be lethal. To give one simple example, in a person who has an extremely high fever approaching the level of lethality, the body metabolism increases to about 100 per cent above normal. By comparison, the metabolism of the body during a marathon race may increase to 2,000 per cent above normal. The final common determinant of success in athletic events is what the muscles can do for you-what strength they can give when it is needed, what power they can achieve in the performance of work, and how long they can continue their activity.

The strength of a muscle is determined mainly by its size, with a maximal contractile force between 3 and 4 kg/cm squared of muscle cross-sectional area. Thus, a man who has enlarged his muscles through an exercise training program will have correspondingly increased muscle strength. An example of muscle strength is a world class weight lifter might have a quadriceps muscle with a cross-sectional area as great as 150 square centimeters. This would translate into a maximal contractile strength of 525 kilograms (or 1155 pounds), with all this force applied to the patellar tendon. Therefore, one can readily understand how it is possible for this tendon at times to be ruptured or actually to be torn from its insertion into the tibia below the knee. Also, when such forces occur in tendons that span a joint, similar forces are applied to the surfaces of the joint or sometimes to ligaments spanning the joints, thus accounting for such happening as displaced cartilages, compression fracture about the joint, and torn ligaments. The holding strength of muscles is about 40 per cent greater than the contractile strength. That is, if a muscle is already contracted and a force then attempts to stretch out the muscle, as occurs when landing after a jump, this requires about 40 per cent more force than can be achieved by a shortening contraction. Therefore, the force of 525 kilograms calculated above for the patellar tendon during muscle contraction becomes 735 kilograms (1617 pounds) during holding contractions. This further compounds the problems of the tendons, joints, and ligaments. It can also lead to internal tearing in the muscle itself. In fact, forceful stretching of a maximally contracted muscle is one of the surest ways to create the highest degree of muscle soreness.

Mechanical work performed by a muscle is the amount of force applied by the muscle multiplied by the distance over which the force is applied.

Another measure of muscle performance is endurance. This, to a great extent, depends on the nutritive support for the muscle, more than anything else on the amount of glycogen that has been stored in the muscle before the period of exercise. A person on a high-carbohydrate diet stores far more glycogen in muscles than a person on either a mixed diet or a high-fat diet. Therefore, endurance is greatly enhanced by a high-carbohydrate diet. When athletes run at speeds typical for the marathon race, their endurance (as measured by the time that they can sustain the race until complete exhaustion) is approximately the following:

	Minutes
High-carbohydrate diet	240
Mixed diet	120
High-fat diet	85

The corresponding amounts of glycogen stored in the muscle before the race started explain these differences. The amounts stored are approximately the following:

	g/kg Muscle
High-carbohydrate diet	40
Mixed-diet	20
High-fat diet	6

Recovery from exhaustive muscle glycogen depletion is not a simple matter. This often requires days, rather than the seconds, minutes, or hours required for recovery. A High-carbohydrate diet, full recovery occurs in about 2 days. Conversely, people on a high-fat, high-protein diet or on no food at all show very little recovery even after as long as 5 days. The messages of this comparison are (1) that it is important for an athlete to have a high-carbohydrate diet before a grueling athletic event and (2) not to participate in exhaustive exercise during the 48 hours preceding the event.

Not all the energy from carbohydrates comes from the stored muscle glycogen. In fact, almost as much glycogen is stored in the liver as in the muscles, and this can be released into the blood in the form of glucose and then taken up by the muscles as an energy source. In addition, glucose solutions given to an athlete to drink during the course of an athletic event can provide as much as 30 to 40 per cent of the energy required during prolonged events. One of the cardinal principles of muscle development during athletic training is the following: Muscles that function under no load, even if they are exercised for hours on end, increase little in strength. At the other extreme, muscles that contract at more than 50 per cent maximal force of contraction will develop strength rapidly even if the contractions are performed only a few times each day. Using this principle, experiments on muscle building have shown that six nearly maximal muscle contractions performed in three sets 3 days a week give approximately optimal increase in muscle strength, without producing chronic muscle fatigue.

In old age, many people become so sedentary that their muscles atrophy tremendously. In these instances, muscle training often increases muscle strength more than 100 per cent.

Normal oxygen consumption for a young man at rest is about 250 ml/min. However, under maximal conditions, this can be increased to approximately the following average levels:

	ml/min
Untrained average male	3600
Athletically trained average male	4000
Male marathon runner	5100

It is clear from this figure, as would be expected, that there is a linear relation. Both oxygen consumption and total pulmonary ventilation increase about 20-fold between the resting state and maximal intensity of exercise in the well-trained athlete.

The important point is that the respiratory system is not normally the most limiting factor in the delivery of oxygen to the muscles during maximal muscle aerobic metabolism. We shall see shortly that the ability of the heart to pump blood to the muscles is usually a greater limiting factor.

The abbreviation for the rate of oxygen usage under maximal aerobic metabolism Vo2 Max. The progressive effect of athletic training on Vo2 Max recorded in a group of subjects beginning at the level of no training and then pursuing the training program for 7 to 13 weeks. In this study, it is surprising that the VO2 Max increased only about 10 per cent. Furthermore, the frequency of training, whether two times or five times per week, had little effect on the increase in VO2 Max.

The oxygen diffusing capacity is a measure of the rate at which oxygen can diffuse from the pulmonary alveoli into the blood. The following are measured values for different diffusing capacities:

	ml/min
Nonathlete at rest	23
Nonathlete during maximal exercise	48
Speed skaters during maximal exercise	64
Swimmers during maximal exercise	71
Oarsman during maximal exercise	80

The most startling fact about these results is that several fold increase in diffusing capacity between the resting state and the state of maximal exercise. This result is mainly from the fact that blood flow through many of the pulmonary capillaries is sluggish or even dormant in the resting state, whereas in maximal exercise, increased blood flow through the lungs causes all the pulmonary capillaries to be at their maximal rates, thus providing a far greater surface area through which oxygen can diffuse into the pulmonary capillary blood. It is also clear from these values that those athletes who require greater amounts of oxygen per minute have higher diffusing capacities. Is this because people with naturally greater diffusing capacities choose these types of sports, or is it because something about the training procedures increases the diffusing capacity? The answer is not known, but it is very likely that training, particularly endurance training, does play an important role.

It is widely known that smoking can decrease an athlete's "wind." This is true for many reasons. First, one effect of nicotine is constriction of the terminal bronchioles of the lungs, which increases the resistance of airflow into and out of the lungs. Second, the irritating effects of the smoke itself cause increased fluid secretion into the bronchial tree as well as some swelling of the epithelial linings. Third, nicotine paralyzes the cilia on the surfaces of the respiratory epithelial cells that normally beat continuously to remove excess fluids and foreign particles from the respiratory passageways. As a result, debris accumulates in the passageways and adds further to the difficulty of breathing. Putting all these factors together, even a light smoker often feels respiratory strain during maximal exercise, and the level of performance may be reduced.

Much more severe are the effects of chronic smoking. There are few chronic smokers in whom some degree of emphysema does not develop. In this disease, the following occur: (1) chronic bronchitis, (2) obstruction of many of the terminal bronchioles, and (3) destruction of many alveolar walls. In severe emphysema, as much as four fifths of the respiratory membrane can be destroyed; then even the slightest exercise can cause respiratory distress. In fact, many such patients cannot even perform the simple feat of walking across the floor of a single room without gasping for breath.

Muscle Blood Flow. A key requirement of cardiovascular function in exercise is to deliver the required oxygen and other nutrients to the exercising muscles. Muscle blood flow can increase a maximum of about 25-fold during the most strenuous exercise. Almost one half this increase in flow results from intramuscular vasodilation. The remaining increase results from multiple factors, the most important of which is probably the moderate increase in arterial blood pressure that occurs in exercise, usually about a 30 per cent increase. The increase in pressure not only forces more blood through the blood vessels but also stretches the walls of the arterioles and further reduces the vascular resistance. Therefore, a 30 per cent increase in blood pressure can often more than double the blood flow.

The normal untrained person can increase cardiac output a little over fourfold, and the well trained athlete can increase output about six fold. Individual marathoners can increase output about seven to eight time's normal resting output. From the foregoing data, it is clear that marathoners can achieve maximal cardiac outputs about 40 per cent greater than those achieved by untrained persons. This result mainly from the fact that the heart chambers of marathoners enlarge about 40 per cent: Along with this enlargement of the chambers, the heart mass also increases 40 per cent or more. Therefore, not only do the skeletal muscles increase during athletic training but the heart does also. However, heart enlargement and increased pumping capacity occur almost entirely in the endurance types, not in the sprint types, of athletic training. Even though the heart of the marathoner is considerably larger than that of the normal person, resting cardiac output is almost exactly the same as that in the normal person. However, this normal cardiac output is achieved by a large stroke volume at a reduced heart rate. Thus, the heart-pumping effectiveness of each heartbeat is 40 to 50 per cent greater in the highly trained athlete than in the untrained person, but there is a corresponding decrease in heart rate at rest.

The stroke volume can increase from 105 to 162 milliliters, an increase of about 50 per cent, whereas the heart rate increases from 50 to 185 beats/min, an increase of 270 per cent. Therefore, the heart rate increase accounts by far for a greater proportion of the increase in cardiac output than does the increase in stroke volume during strenuous exercise. The stroke volume normally reaches its maximum by the time the cardiac output has increased only halfway to its maximum. Any further increase in cardiac output must occur by increasing the heart rate. For this reason, it is frequently stated that the level of athletic performance that can be achieved by the marathoner mainly depends on the performance capability of his or her heart, because this is the most limiting link in the delivery of adequate oxygen to the exercising muscles. Therefore, the 40 per cent greater cardiac output that the marathoner can achieve over the average untrained male is probably the single most important physiologic benefit of the marathoner's training program.

Effect of heart disease and old age on athletic performance. Because of the critical limitation that the cardiovascular system places on maximal performance in endurance athletics. One can readily understand that any type of heart disease that reduces maximal cardiac output will cause an almost corresponding decrease in achievable total body muscle power. Therefore, a person with congestive heart failure frequently has difficulty achieving even the muscle power required to climb out of bed, much less to walk across the floor.

The maximal cardiac output of an older person also decreases considerably. There is as much as a 50 per cent decrease between age 18 and age 80. Also, there is even more decrease in maximal breathing capacity. For these reasons, as well as reduced skeletal muscle mass, the maximal achievable muscle power is greatly reduced in old age.

Body Heat in Exercise

Almost all the energy released by the body's metabolism of nutrients is eventually converted into heat. This applies even to the energy that causes muscle contraction for the following reasons: First, the maximal efficiency for conversion of nutrient energy into muscle work, even under the best of conditions, is only 20 to 25 per cent; the remainder of the nutrient energy is converted into heat during the course of the intracellular chemical reactions. Second, almost all the energy that does go into creating muscle work still becomes body heat because all but a small portion of this energy is used for (1) overcoming viscous resistance to the movement of the muscles and joints, and (2) overcoming the friction of the blood flowing through the blood vessels.

Now, recognizing that the oxygen consumption by the body can increase as much as 20-fold in the well-trained athlete and that the amount of heat liberated in the body is almost exactly proportional to the oxygen consumption, one quickly realizes that tremendous amounts of heat are injected into the internal body tissues when performing endurance athletic events. Next, with a vast rate of heat flow into the body, on a very hot and humid day so that the sweating mechanism cannot eliminate the heat, an intolerable and even lethal condition called heatstroke can easily develop in the athlete.

During endurance athletics even under normal environmental conditions the body temperature often rises from its normal level of 98.6 to 102 or 103 F (37 to 40 C). With very hot and humid conditions or excess clothing, the body temperature can easily rise to 106 to 108 F (41 to 42 C). At this level, the elevated temperature itself becomes destructive to tissue cells, especially the brain cells. When this happens, multiple symptoms begin to appear, including extreme weakness, exhaustion, headache, dizziness, nausea, profuse sweating, confusion, staggering gait, collapse, and unconsciousness.

This whole complex is called heatstroke, and failure to treat it immediately can lead to death. In fact, even though the person has stopped exercising, the temperature does not easily decrease by itself. One of the reasons for this is that at these high temperatures, the temperature-regulating mechanism itself fails. A second reason is that in heatstroke, the very high body temperature itself approximately doubles the rate of all intracellular chemical reactions, thus liberating still more heat.

The treatment of heatstroke is to reduce the body temperature as rapidly as possible. The most practical way to do this is to remove all clothing, maintain a spray of cool water on all surfaces of the body or continually sponge the body, blow air over the body with a fan, or total immersion of the body in water containing a mush of crushed ice if available.

As much as a 5 to 10 pound weight loss has been recorded in athletes in a period of 1 hour during endurance athletic event under hot and humid condition. Essentially all this weight loss results from loss of sweat. Loss of enough sweat to decrease body weight only 3 per cent can significantly diminish a person's performance, and a 5 to 10 per cent rapid decrease in weight can often be serious, leading to muscle cramps, nausea, and other effects. Therefore, it is essential to replace fluid as it is lost. A person must replace sodium chloride and potassium. As a consequence of these findings, some of the supplemental fluids for athletics contain properly proportioned amounts of potassium along with sodium, usually in the form of fruit juices or other supplemental fluids.

Multiple studies have now shown that people who maintain appropriate body fitness, using regimens of exercise and weight control, have the additional benefit of prolonged life. Especially between the ages of 50 and 70, studies have shown mortality to be three times less in the fit people than in the least fit.

Why does body fitness prolong life? The following are the two most evident reasons. First body fitness and weight control greatly reduce cardiovascular disease. This results from (1) maintenance of moderately lower blood pressure and (2) reduced blood cholesterol and low-density lipoprotein (LDL) along with increased high-density lipoprotein (HDL). As pointed out earlier, these changes all work together to reduce the number of heart attacks and brain strokes.

Second, and perhaps equally important, the athletically fit person has more bodily reserve to call on when he or she does become sick. For instance, an 80-year-old nonfat person may have a respiratory system that limits oxygen delivery to the tissues to no more than 1 L/min; this means a respiratory reserve of no more than threefold to fourfold. However, an athletically fit old person may have twice as much reserve. This is especially important in preserving life when the older person develops condition such as pneumonia that can rapidly require all available respiratory reserve. In addition, the ability to increase cardiac output in times of need (the "cardiac reserve") is often 50 per cent greater in the athletically fit old person than in the nonfat person.

CHAPTER XXII:

Bone Density

On Sept. 24 2008 I had my bone density measured, the results were amazing. At the age of 66 I have the bone density of a 30 year old.

T-Score o.47 (106%) average population score %

Z-Score (119%) 60 year old population score %

These results were obtained with flexing and massaging. I will explain how the bone density changed within my body. Remember how sore and painful my feet were. This was because the bones were weak and causing these results.

Bone health fact: It is actually possible to help reverse bone loss and strengthen bones. The physiology of calcium and phosphate metabolism in the formation of bone. The regulation of vitamin D, parathyroid hormone (PTH), and calcitonin are all closely related. Extra cellular (fluid outside the cell) calcium ion concentration is determined by the interplay of calcium absorption from the intestine, renal excretion of calcium, and bone uptake and release of calcium, each of which is regulated by the hormones as just noted.

An important feature of extracellular calcium regulation is that only about 0.1 per cent of the total body calcium is in the extracellular fluid, about 1 per cent is in the cells, and the rest is stored in bones. Therefore, the bones can serve as large reservoirs, releasing calcium when extracellular fluid concentration decreases. This greatly decreases bone mineralization causing the bone density to become weaker.

The usual rates of intake are about 1000 mg/day each for calcium and phosphorus, about the amounts in 1 liter of milk (don't drink milk). This amount should be taken with supplements for a healthy diet. Vitamin D promotes calcium absorption by the intestines. When calcium concentration is low, this reabsorption is great, so that almost no calcium is lost in the urine.

A Harvard Nurses study stated Post-menopausal women in America who consume calcium rich dairy products have over three times more osteoporosis than those who do not. This is because milk products have about 10 times more calcium than magnesium. Rates of osteoporosis are lowest in cultures where the ratio of calcium to magnesium is between 2 parts calcium to 3 parts magnesium.

Stop drinking soft drinks! They are high in phosphoric acid and sugar, making these drinks highly acidic. Calcium is the main mineral the body uses to neutralize acid. So phosphoric acid depletes calcium levels by causing it to be pulled from the bone.

A diet high in meat and carbohydrates, with few greens or fruit will be highly acidic. This causes the body to utilize calcium to neutralize the acids.

Bone is composed of a tough organic matrix that is greatly strengthened by deposits of calcium salts. Average compact bone contains by weight about 30 per cent matrix and 70 per cent salts. The organic matrix of bone is 90 to 95 per cent collagen fiber, and the remainder is ground substance. The collagen fiber gives the tissue powerful tensile strength. The crystalline salts deposited in the organic matrix of bone are composed principally of calcium and phosphate. The collagen fibers of bone, like those of tendons, have great tensile strength, where as the calcium salts have great compressional strength. These combined properties plus the degree of bondage between the collagen fibers and the crystals provide a bony structure that has both extreme tensile strength and extreme compressional strength.

The rise in calcium concentration for the intracellular fluid is caused by the effect of parathyroid hormone. PTH increase calcium and phosphate absorption from the bone. PTH causes removal of bone salts from the bone matrix and along the bone surface causing more damage to the density of the bone.

Bone contains such great amounts of calcium in comparison with the total amount in all the extra cellular fluids (about 1000 times as much) that even when PTH causes a great rise in calcium concentration in the fluids, it is impossible to discern any immediate effect on the bones. Prolonged administration or secretion of PTH-over a period of many months or years-finally results in very evident absorption in all the bones and even development of large cavities which fill with large multinucleated osteoclasts.

Bone resorption is the process by which osteoclasts break down and release the minerals, resulting in a transfer of calcium from bone fluid to the blood. Bone resorption can also be the result of disuse and the lack of stimulus for bone maintenance. Astronauts, for instance will undergo a certain amount of bone resorption due to the lack of gravity, providing the proper stimulus for bone maintenance. Calcium sensing receptors in the parathyroid gland monitor calcium levels in the extra cellular fluid. Low levels of calcium stimulate the release of parathyroid hormone. PTH also increases the number activity of osteoclasts to release calcium from bone, and thus stimulates bone resorption. High levels of calcium in the blood leads to decreased PTH, decreasing the number and activity of osteoclasts, resulting in less or no bone resorption. It is very important that you get that right amount of calcium and magnesium in your diet.

Bones are living tissues that must be constantly rebuilt via a two part process. First, cells called osteoclasts clear old minerals out of bone tissue that has become weak and mottled, and carry it into the blood. Next, osteoblasts deposit new minerals and collagen back into the bone.

Osteoclast and osteoblasts are activated by the parathyroid hormone which encourages osteoclasts to pull calcium from the bones. Calcitonin is the hormone that stimulates osteoblasts to deposit calcium into the bones. When we lack magnesium, the balance between PTH and calcitonin tilts too far toward PTH. This results in excessive stimulation of osteoclasts, which causes net bone loss. Increasing magnesium is the natural way to correct this. Studies also show that magnesium supplements, even when used without calcium increased bone density.

Bone is continually being deposited by osteoblasts, and it is continually being absorbed where osteoclasts are active. Osteoblasts are found on the outer surfaces of the bone and in the bone cavities. A small amount of osteoblastic activity occurs continually in all living bones (on about 4 per cent of all surfaces at any given time in an adult), so that at least some new bone is being formed constantly. The osteoclasts are normally active on less than 1 per cent of the bone surfaces of an adult.

Normally, except in growing bones, the rate of bone deposition and absorption are equal to each other, so that the total mass of bone remains constant. Osteoclasts usually exist in small but concentrated masses, and once a mass of osteoclasts begins to develop, it usually eats away at the bone for about 3 weeks, creating a tunnel that ranges in diameter from 0.2 to 1 millimeter and is several millimeters long. At the end of this time, the osteoclasts disappear and the tunnel is invaded by osteoblasts instead; then new bone begins to develop. Bone deposition then continues for several months, until the tunnel is filled.

The continual deposition and absorption of bone have several physiologically important functions. First, bone ordinarily adjusts it strength (increased bone density) in proportion to the degree of bone stress. Consequently, bones thicken when subjected to heavy loads. (When using flexing and deep massaging, you applied stress to the bone, causing this affect. At the age of 66 or older, you can apply pressure to the bone which will increase the density of the bone. That is why I have the bone density of a 30 year old. You can obtain the same results without the use of any drugs by using my method of flexing and messaging.) Second, even the shape of the bone can be rearranged for proper support of mechanical forces by deposition and absorption of bone in accordance with stress patterns. Third, because old bone becomes relatively brittle and weak, a new organic matrix is needed as the old organic matrix degenerates. In this manner, the normal toughness of bone is maintained.

Bone is deposited in proportion to the compressional load that the bone must carry. For instance, the bones of athletes become considerably heavier than those of nonathletes. Also, if a person has one leg in a cast but continues to walk on the opposite leg, the bone of the leg in the cast becomes thin and as much as 30 per cent decalcified within a few weeks, whereas the opposite bone remains thick and normally calcified. Therefore, continual physical stress stimulates osteoblastic deposition and calcification of bone. (Again, all these results can be obtained with flexing and massaging.) You can obtain these results at any age. When flexing and massaging the muscle, you are also applying pressure to the bones this will also strengthen the bones. This is very important, if you have a sore spot in the bone; you should massage these spots until the soreness subsides. This may happen the first time you message the area or it may take several times until the pain subsides. The constant pressure applied to the bone will stimulate the osteoprogenitor cells, which are bone stem cells further increasing bone strength.

Several studies have shown that taking calcium and vitamin D helps the elderly have fewer of the falls and fractures that can lead to prolonged hospitalization and even death. For example, in one study of 389 men and women over age 65 who took 500 milligrams of calcium and 700 IU of vitamin D, fractures decreased by 58 percent. "The jury is in," says Dr. Heaney. "These supplements definitely reduce fracture risk."

"Why osteoporosis drugs actually make your bones weak and brittle. Recent studies have linked these drugs to osteonecrosis of the jaw, an incurable condition where the bone in the jaw actually dies!" stated M.D. Susan Lark.

Some 2,400 people have developed this devastating condition, and many are suing the drug companies. In response, one of the drug companies issued a press release saying that these cases "do not necessarily indicate causality." This isn't true. Here's why bisphosphonate drugs can harm your bones. Your bones keep renewing themselves throughout your life, with older, weaker bone cells being replaced by younger, stronger ones. This happens because two special cells called osteoclasts and osteoblasts. The osteoclasts break down old bone and remove it, and then the osteoblasts build new bone. Bisphosphonate drugs work by disabling the osteoclasts so that they stop breaking down your old bone. But these drugs do nothing to build new bone. Even though your bones become denser, that density is made up of old, weak, brittle bone tissue.

So why did these cases of bone death occur in the jaw and not other bones? It's a medical fact that the orthoclase/osteopath cycle moves a lot faster in the jaw than it does in the other bones of the body. That is why the bone changes caused by these drugs would occur in the jaw first.

It's been a little over 10 years since the introduction of bisphosphonate drugs. In the next 10 years we will start seeing cases of bone death in the legs, arms, and hips. Again with flexing and messaging you can avoid these problems.

Prunes build stronger bones. If someone asked you what to eat for strong bones, it's unlikely that prunes would top your list. But antioxidants in prunes (dried plums) increase bone formation in animals. This is stated in a new test at the University Oklahoma. Researchers suggest that eating prunes could benefit people at risk of osteoporosis. Previous research found that feeding prunes to animals could both prevent and reverse bone loss, and those post-menopausal women who ate 3.5 ounces a day (about 10 prunes) showed signs of improved bone mineral density. Prunes have more protective antioxidants than any other fruit.

CHAPTER XXIII:
Stem Cells Regeneration

In the past two years, the time I been writing my book. A lot of interesting things have happened. My thoughts of increasing muscle to prolong life are the number one method in this process. Major universities are spending millions of dollars on this process and have not yet figured out how to prolong life by increasing muscle mass. By reading my book you are headed in the right direction to live a longer and healthy life.

At the present time I am corresponding with Michael Rae; who works for Aubrey de Grey: The number one person on the extension of life. They show much interest in what I am doing. They are doing all their research on mice and I am doing all my research on my own body. The results are very similar. I will explain these results to you.

Fat cells are very important in the extension of life. Fat cells protect vital organs, store fuel and energy in case food gets scarce, make hormones work and control chemicals that regulate brain function, the immune system and metabolism. Without fat cells life would be impossible.

Scientists are delving ever-deeper into the mysteries of fat cells and discovering more and more about the functions of these cells. The Institute for Advanced Reconstruction and the Plastic Surgery Center in New Jersey research shows that a glob of fat contains not only adipocytes (mature, or adult, fat cells) but also preadipocytes (immature fat cells), and is a source of adult stem cells (precursor cells that have the potential to develop in various cells and tissues).

There is also evidence that fat is stimulated by certain chemicals in the body. One of these is insulin growth factor, or IGF (Growth Hormone). IGFs are part of a complex system that cells use to communicate with their physiologic environment. The IGF axis has been shown to play roles in the promotion of cell production and the restraint of cell death. Factors that are known to cause variation in the levels of IGF include age, exercise status, stress levels, nutrition level and body mass index. Almost every cell in the human body is affect by IGF, especially cells in muscle, cartilage, bone, liver, kidney, nerves, skin, and lungs. In addition to the insulin-like effects they can also regulate cell growth and development, especially in nerve cells, as well as cellular DNA synthesis.

Fat is a source of stem cells which have the potential to develop into various kinds of cells and tissues. These stem cells can become any type of cell-bone cells, fat cells, and muscle cells. It all depends on the induction that you use for them. By using flexing and massaging you can stimulate these cells to regenerate muscle, bone, cartilage and skin cells. An example is when the muscle cells turn to fat and fiber. The fats cells which contain these stem cells can produce more muscle cell. By stimulating the cells with flexing and massaging; this increase of muscle mass will prolong life by returning the muscle back to the original 50% mark.

Another example about my bone density is a bone health fact. It's actually possible to help reverse bone loss and strengthen bones. On Sept 24, I had my bone density measured. The result where amazing, my T-score was .47. This is the score of a 30 year old. This result was obtained by flexing and messaging. I no longer worry about thinning bones, vertebral or hip fracture, and osteoporosis. You can obtain the same results. This process will take a few years before you obtain similar results. When I talked about foot massage and flexing; my feet where very sore and painful. After four years, my feet were pain free, because I increased the bone density. You must flex your feet throughout the day to obtain these results. After your feet become pain free; you will flex your feet only a few times a day. Other results in the book where facial massage, cartilage repair in the knee, and ligament repair in the rotator cup. All these results were obtained with flexing and massaging.

Body composition analysis is about how the human body is composed of bone, muscle, internal organs, water, and adipose tissue (fat tissue). A variety of techniques have been developed to evaluate the total body fat percentage. Hydrostatic Body Fat Testing is referred to as the gold standard, or the method by which all other methods measure their own accuracy. On Sept. 24, 2008 I had this procedure done. These are the result.

Body Fat:
Percentage:	16.7
Weight of Body Fat (lb):	32.6
Lean Body Mass:	
Lean Body Mass Percentage:	83.4%
Weight of Lean Body Mass (lb):	163
Total Weight of Body (lb):	195.6
Current Status and Goals	

According to my age group (60+) and my percent of fat 16.7% placing me at the 85% percentile with a rating of

"Healthy Range".This number also places me in the age group (40+) at 75% percentile with a rating of "Healthy Range". I said throughout the book that I felt and perform like a forty year old.This is some scientific data proving this statement.

At the age of sixty my body weight was 230 lbs. I did a lot of research (all the information in my book) with a healthy diet and doing exercising with flexing and messaging. I lost 35 lbs. Because I increased my muscle mass, I was able to burn more calories. You can do all these procedures while sitting down watching TV.You will increase your muscle mass and with the added muscle mass you will burn more calories. With the increase in muscle mass you will feel healthy and younger.You will be doing things you never thought possible at your age. One example is that I started running again at the age of sixty five.

I discovered that when the muscle turned to fat tissue and fiber the muscle was no longer a solid mass. It had holes or empty spaces within the muscle tissue. I was pulling a heavy object and my knee joints were slipping from the force, because lack of muscle mass. I physically discovered the lack of muscle that was replaced by fat tissue and fiber. By stimulating the muscle you make the muscle a solid, larger mass. When muscles turns to fat tissue/fat cells (the cells containing stem cells), the muscle can be stimulated (flexing and massaging). This change the fat cells back to muscle mass.

My muscles are larger and more ripped (muscles with full striation). This process is regeneration of muscle mass and can be used to increase your life span. Man hadn't discovered this process until now. I can mold my muscles any way that I want. I can control the muscle mass making the muscle larger.

Stem cells which are found in the fat cells can become any type of cell. The stem cells became more muscle cells in my case. It all depends on the induction that you use for them. Stem cells are likely to stimulate cell growth and inhibit cell death. There is an intimate relationship between fat tissue in the body and insulin production of IGF. These growth hormones promote synthesis of new protein. In this case it is more muscle mass. At the same time the stem cells conserved the proteins already present in the cell causing the muscle to grow. By stimulating these cells, they turn into more muscle mass instead of more fats cells. The example of an 80 year old person has to turn 30 pounds of fat cells (this equals 30 percent muscle mass) back into 30 pounds of muscle. Losing muscle mass is one of the leading causes of death. Death ordinarily ensues when the proteins (muscle mass) of the body have been depleted to about 50 percent their normal level.

Losing muscle mass also causes a decline in the number of mitochondria. You have two thousand mitochondrion per cell. Every cell contains thousands of strands of mitochondrial DNA. The function and dysfunction of the mitochondria serves as the backbone for one of the major theories of aging. Keeping the muscle mass at a constant level will keep the mitochondria from aging. Mitochondria sustain some type of damage as the muscle turns into fat cells. Antioxidants are important factors in controlling mitochondria damage. Losing mitochondria as you lose muscle mass is a major cause of glycosylation causing even more damage to cells, tissues, and organs of the body.

At the age of 60, people would make comments on how I walked because it looked so painful. I spent thousands of dollars on my feet with no results. At the age of 65 I'm running. I no longer have problems with my feet, because of flexing and massage.

I get some of my best workouts while watching TV at night. The growth of muscle mass will be noticed within a few months. The overall result will take years to reach. It took five years before I could run. I turned 24 pounds of fiber and fat tissue back into muscle with flexing and massaging. This procedure will have to be performed the rest of my life, for 150 years or longer to maintain these results. After six years smaller muscles are at full strength and size. The larger muscles are still growing and increasing in strength. The process takes time. All of these results you can obtain. You can achieve increased bone density, strengthened ligaments, increased muscle mass and repaired cartilage. These are all examples of regeneration, with flexing and massaging. You can live a longer and healthier life with Extension of Life: Self Healing.

CHAPTER XXIV:
Restless Leg Syndrome

Who wouldn't give practically anything to be able to sleep normal again, without any restless leg syndrome? I know the answer. That is what I am going to teach you a way that will enable you to sleep normal again without the pain and discomfort you thought were inevitable.

It would be unusual for anyone reading this claim to not be a little skeptical. So rest assured that what you will read here is based on my own personal experience and a lot of knowledge accumulated over many years. I have put the technique I am going to share with you into practice, and I am here to tell you that it works.

Why suffer through sleepless nights caused by restless legs when you don't have to? I will show you how to get major relief from your restless legs, eliminate sleepless night, dramatically improve your quality of sleep and wake up feeling rested and super-refreshed.

The exact cause of restless legs syndrome is not known. Restless legs syndrome can be a primary or a secondary condition. Primary restless leg syndrome is the main form of the disease. No one is sure what causes primary restless legs syndrome. There is currently no cure for primary restless leg syndrome. I will show you how to get major relief from restless leg syndrome. The first time you try this there will be instant relief. Faster than any other treatment. In fact, I challenge you to find a faster remedy.

I will explain why I can make this statement. When you read the rest of this article it will explain why I am so confident these statements are correct. I would love to tell you I am a genius, but I really found it by accident. The secret cure for restless leg syndrome is easy, available and inexpensive.

At an early age I had secondary restless leg syndrome. At the age of 55 it turned into primary restless leg syndrome, also at this age I developed major feet problems. So my Doctor gave me a non narcotic pain medicine for my foot pain. He also give me carbi/levodopa for my RLS. I took my RLS pills at night and I noticed that they didn't work. But when I took my pain medicine for my feet at night, my RLS pain disappeared. So I could control my RLS with my pain medicine. I just made my major discovery on how to control RLS. I didn't think this was a big deal. I was pain free from RLS for the last ten years and my Doctor thinks I use this medicine for my foot pain.

On 1/8/08 I figured out how important this discovery was. I met Robert and he had a sleeping problem. He didn't explain his sleeping problem very well to me. I told him to try Benadryl. He did. It wired him and he didn't sleep the whole night. I talked to him the next day and I felt really bad about him not sleeping. So we talked about his sleeping problems. He said that he was born with RLS. When he was a child he would go to bed at night and lie there the whole night. He didn't know that people slept at night. He had this sleeping problem for 67 years, only sleeping a few minutes each night. He spent thousands of dollars trying to fix his RLS problem. He was a patient for Einstein Medical Institute of New York taking the newest medication for RLS. None of these medications worked. He was one of the first patients to try Ropinirole before it was approved by U.S. Food and Drug Administration and it didn't work. He was an individual patient for the doctor who developed these drugs. He also went to a sleeping expert to help him sleep and that didn't work. I told him I had RLS that I solved my problem by taking my pain medication. So, I gave him a few of my pills and told him to try them. He took one pill at 2 o clock PM and another just before bed time. He slept for four hours the first time he tried this drug. He was pain free for several hours and could sit and watch television without the discomfort of RLS. So you might be thinking he only slept for four hours. If your medicine is so great why didn't he sleep the whole night? Remember he was pain free for the first time in his life and he slept for four hours. The reason he didn't sleep longer was because he took only one pill. The next experiment by Robert included taking three pills two hours before bed time and he is sleeping the whole night. He stated that this was the greatest discovery in his life. He was free of RLS for the first time in his life.

I have taken this medication for ten years. When I first started taking this mediation. I took two pills every six hours, after six hours the mediation would wear off. Several times I tried to stop taking this medication but within ten hours the RLS would return. I figured that the best result for me is to take three pills when I wake up in the morning and three pills two hours before I go to sleep. If I worked in the yard for several hours or walked eighteen holes of golf this would stir up my RLS and I would have to take two pills to calm it down. I really didn't know how important my medication was until I lost it on a trip to Mexico. Sitting on the plane for several hours I needed my medication, putting it back in my travel bag it dropped on the floor. That night we went to a fiesta had a few drinks and ate a lot. When I came back to the room to take my pills and then go to sleep. I couldn't find my mediation. I was in for a long night. My leg became very uncomfortable tossing and turning all night. I tried taking several Advil and Ibuprofen but they didn't work. I couldn't get my medication until the airport was open at 9 o clock in the morning. That was the most uncomfortable might I ever had in my life. That's when I realized how important my medication was for my RLS. When taking this medication you have to figure out how many pills to take. Two pills work for only six hours and three pills work for twelve hour, in my case. You have to figure out how many pills you need to take for yourself. Never take more than three pills at a time.

This medication is a prescription drug. Tell your Doctor you read this article and you would like to relieve your RLS by taking TRAMADOL. Repeated doses of this drug can cure all our ills. You will feel better as long as you keep taking the drug. This drug will not lead to addiction, because it is non narcotic and you won't develop a tolerance to this drug. It will cure the spasms which cause discomfort and fatigue of RLS and then you will finally get a full night sleep.

This publication contains the opinions and ideas of its author. It is intended to provide helpful material on the subject addressed in this book. It is sold with the understanding that the author is not engaged in rendering medical, health, or any other kind of personal professional services in the book. The reader should consult his or her medical, health, or other competent professional before adopting any of the suggestions of this book. The author specifically disclaims any and all responsibility for liability or injury which is incurred as a consequence of the use of any of the contents in this book.

CHAPTER XXV:
The External Signals That Control Regeneration

A significant hurdle to this use and most uses of stem cells is that scientists do not yet fully understand the signals that turn specific gene on and off to influence the differentiation (specialized cells, like muscles cells) of the stem cell. Could I have discovered this signal?

Stem cells have the remarkable potential to develop into many different cell types in the body. Serving as a sort of repair system for the body, they can divide without limit to replenish other cells. When a stem cell divides, each new cell has the potential to either remain a stem cell or become another type of cell (differentiation) with a more specialized function, such as a muscle cell, a red blood cell, or a brain cell.

Scientists primarily work with two kinds of stem cells from animals and humans: Embryonic stem cell and adult stem cell. We will only concentrate on adult stem cell, which are found in the human body.

Research on stem cells is advancing knowledge about how an organism develops from a single cell and how healthy cells replace damaged cells in adult organisms. This promising area of science is also leading scientists to investigate the possibility of cell-based therapies to treat disease or repair tissues and organs, which are often referred to as regenerative medicine.

Stem cells have two important characteristics that distinguish them from other types of cells. First, they are unspecialized cells that renew themselves for long periods through cell division. The second is that under certain physiologic or experimental conditions, they can be induced to become cells with special functions such as the beating cells of the heart muscle, formation of increase muscle mass or increasing bone density.

Stem cells differ from other kinds of cells in the body. All stem cells-regardless of their source-have three general properties: They are capable of diving and renewing themselves for long periods; they are unspecialized; and they can give rise to specialized cell types.

What are the factors in living organisms that normally regulate stem cell proliferation and self-renewal? Discovering the answer to these questions may make it possible to understand how cell proliferation is regulated during the abnormal cell division that leads to cancer. Stem cells are capable of dividing and renewing themselves for long periods. When cells replicate themselves many times over it is called proliferation. A starting population of stem cells that proliferates can yield millions of cells.

An important area of research is understanding the signals in a mature organism that cause a stem cell population to proliferate and remain unspecialized until the cells are needed for repair of a specific tissue. Such information is critical for scientists to be able to control these stem cells. Stem cells can give rise to specialized cells. When unspecialized stem cells give rise to specialized cells, the process is called differentiation. Scientists are just beginning to understand the signals inside and outside cells that trigger stem cell differentiation. The internal signals are controlled by a cell's genes. The external signals for cell differentiation include chemicals secreted by other cells, or physical contact with neighboring cells. Scientists haven't been able to figure out this signal at the present time. If a specific set of signals can be identified that will promote differentiation into specific cell types with these signals man could control stem cell differentiation. There by growing cells of tissues that can be used for specific purpose.

Therefore, many questions about stem cell differentiation remain. For example, are the internal and external signals for cell differentiation similar for all kinds of stem cell? Can specific set of signals be identified that promote differentiation into specific cell types? Addressing these questions is critical because the answers may lead scientist to find new ways of controlling stem cell differentiation. Adult stem cells typically generate the cell types of the tissue in which they reside. Over the last several years have raised the possibility that stem cells from one tissue may be able to give rise to cell types of a completely different tissue.

Adult stem cells have been identified in many organs and tissues. One important point to understand about adult stem cells is that there are a very small number of stem cells in each tissue. Stem cells are thought to reside in a specific area of each tissue where they may remain quiescent (non-dividing) for many years until they are activated by disease, tissue injury, or are stimulated by physical contact (flexing and massaging). The adult tissues reported to contain stem cells include brain, bone, bone marrow, blood vessels, skeletal muscle, skin and liver. A single adult stem cell should be able to generate a line of genetically identical cells-known as a clone-which then gives rise to all the appropriate differentiated cell types of the tissue. Scientists have been able to demonstrate that individual adult stem cell clones have the ability to repopulate tissues in a living animal (my own body). Adult stem cells can divide for a long period and can give rise to mature cell types that have characteristic shapes and specialized structures and functions of a particular tissue. An adult stem cell is an undifferentiated cell found among differentiated cells in a tissue or organ, can renew itself, and can differentiate to yield the major specialized cell types of the tissue or organ.

The primary role of adult stem cells in a living organism are to maintain and repair the tissue in which they are found, (example; muscle turns to fat cells and fiber, with flexing and massaging, you can change these materials back into the original muscle mass, and you can make the muscle even larger with this process) through the use of the stem cells. Bone marrow stromal cells (stem cells) give rise to a variety of cell types: Bone cell, cartilage cells, fat cells, and other kinds of connective tissue cells such as those in tendons, which can repair these tissues.

If a specific set of signals can be identified that will promote differentiation into specific cell types. With these signals man can control stem cell differentiation. There by growing cells or tissues that can be used for human repair.

I have discovered this signal which is flexing and massaging which will promote differentiation into specific cell types. The following examples will prove this statement. By using flexing and massaging I stimulated the muscle stem cells to regenerate more muscle mass. I have the muscle mass of a forty year old. I stimulated the bone to regenerate more bone which increased the bone density; I have the bone density of a thirty year old. The torn cartilage in my knee and torn rotator cup was repaired with stem cells regenerating more cartilage and connective tissue. Fewer wrinkles on my face and neck regenerating collagen in the skin. With flexing and massaging we are stimulating the stem cell to repair and strength the cells, tissues, and organs of our body.

I no longer have a fear of aging with time as my body continues to get younger with flexing and massaging. I have the bone density of a thirty year old and the muscle mass of a forty year old. My body continue to gain more muscle mass and is getting stronger as it ages. I no longer have the aches and pain that comes with aging. I am sharing this information with others in hopes that they can obtain these same results.

CHAPTER XXVI:

Drug Industry

Have you ever noticed the pens, and other trinkets at your doctor's office? Chances are, they were labeled with the brand name of the prescription drug company. The pharmaceutical industry has been giving these types of small gifts to doctors for years, in hopes of raising physician's awareness of their medications. This relationship has raised increasing concerns that these marketing tactics are influencing physicians' decisions on the drugs they prescribe.

The Pharmaceutical Research and Manufacturers of America, the industry's trade group, recently acknowledged that branded trinkets "are not based on informing (physician) about medical and scientific issues." It instituted a voluntary ban on drug companies giving gifts to doctors.

Representatives from drug companies often leave samples of brand-name medications for doctors to dispense. Because only heavily promoted-and often the most expensive-drugs are sampled in most cases, patients must pay for refills at prices significantly higher than a generic drug of similar efficacy.

A study published last year in Medical Care, showed that out-of-pocket cost for prescription drugs increased 47 percent for patients who received free medications to try, when compared with those who were not offered such samples.

Medication sampling accounts for $16 billion a year, or half the pharmaceutical industry's marketing budget. Numerous studies have shown that physicians who had access to samples tended to give more expensive medications, which is a concern when prescription drugs cost $227.5 billion annually.

Research shows that many doctors rely more on the pharmaceutical industry's own information about a medication than on checking independent sources for evaluation of the drug. Only 26 percent of physicians used medical journals. Also, programs where representatives recommend cheaper, but equally effective, generic drugs to doctors need to be better funded and promoted.

Courses doctors must take are funded in large part by the drug industry and that subsidy comes at a price. By allowing industry funding, doctors tend to receive educational lectures that require expensive treatments and indirectly increase the use of the funder's drug. As the practice of free medication sampling continues. The pharmaceutical industry will continue to help direct your doctor's prescribing pen.

Index